Health Professionals
Style Manual

About the Authors

Shirley H. Fondiller, EdD, RN, FAAN, an internationally known journalist, educator, and historian, is cofounder and principal of Publishing for Health Dimensions (*phd*), an editorial service for nurses and health professionals. She has presented workshops on writing for publication and written extensively on the topic, including *The Writer's Workbook* (1999), a hands-on resource for beginning authors in the health field. Dr. Fondiller has prepared monographs for leading private foundations, historiographies of influential national organizations, and scripts for the broadcast media.

Barbara J. Nerone, APR, has a broad background in the communications field. She served as executive editor of *Imprint*, the magazine of the National Student Nurses Association, and has written and edited articles for nursing journals and publications of national associations and service agencies. Ms. Nerone has spoken widely on the subjects of professional writing, publishing, and public relations and taught writing and grammar for business professionals. She is cofounder and principal of Publishing for Health Dimensions (*phd*).

Health Professionals Style Manual

Shirley Fondiller, EdD, RN, FAAN
Barbara J. Nerone, APR

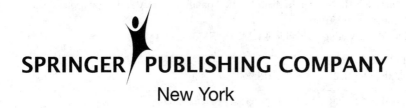

SPRINGER PUBLISHING COMPANY
New York

Springer Publishing Company, LLC
11 West 42nd Street
New York, NY 10036

Acquisitions Editor: Sally J. Barhydt
Managing Editor: Mary Ann McLaughlin
Production Editor: Emily Johnston
Cover design: Mimi Flow
Composition: Apex Covantage

06 07 08 09 10/ 5 4 3 2 1

Library of Congress Cataloging-in-Publication Data

Fondiller, Shirley H.
Health professionals style manual / Shirley Fondiller, Barbara J. Nerone.
     p. ; cm.
  Rev. ed. of: Health professionals stylebook, c1993.
  Includes bibliographical references and index.
  ISBN 0–8261–0207–7   1. Medical writing—Handbooks,
manuals, etc. I. Nerone, Barbara J. II. Fondiller, Shirley H. Health professionals
stylebook. III. Title.
[DNLM: 1. Writing—Handbooks. WZ 29 F673h 2006]

R119.F66 2006
808′.06661—dc22   2006018588

Printed in the United States of America by Bang Printing

Contents

Preface

Some years ago, David Lambuth, the colorful professor of English at Dartmouth College, communicated his passion for precise expression to his students over a long career in teaching. In a pithy handbook on writing that became a classic in the field, he wrote that *good writing* must be clear, vivid, and moving. Lambuth also described *bad writing,* and in his own inimitable style characterized it as faulty and foolish, muddy and mucky, sloppy and sleazy!

Whether you are required to write a class paper or a thesis, submitting a manuscript for publication in a professional journal or making a conference presentation, or simply sending a memo to your staff or colleagues, the ability to write effectively is a critical skill. The *Health Professionals Style Manual* will provide you with basic guidelines and tips about writing clearly and correctly, but nothing can substitute for sitting down and putting your thoughts in a logical and coherent form. As you begin the process, remember that the person who thinks clearly should write clearly, ensuring that every word contributes to conveying your information concisely. Acquiring this skill means fortifying yourself with the essential ingredients: developing an adequate vocabulary and a knowledge of proper usage. Writers, therefore, must read widely and intelligently.

WHAT YOU WILL FIND IN THIS BOOK

The five chapters of the *Style Manual* cover writing style, whether formal or informal; tips on the "art" of effective writing; specific tips and pitfalls in language usage presented in a convenient alphabetical format; the importance of avoiding redundancy and euphemisms; and the advantages that computers and specialized software give the 21st-century writer. Reference material has been organized in Appendixes A to F, in which you will find lists of common abbreviations and acronyms, commonly misspelled words, correct use of prefixes and suffixes, proofreader's marks, valuable electronic resources, and guidelines on referencing. Following the appendices, we provide References for Further Reading. We consider this to be *your* guide for references. The works cited are those we consider the best in the writing business and the most helpful in providing you with supplementary information.

In preparing the *Style Manual,* our approach was to examine existing books for their relevance, cull or modify the most useful material, pull together information for health professionals not found elsewhere, and put it all in one handy reference. We knew that some duplication with other books would be necessary but for emphasis only. From the outset, we searched contemporary style manuals of respected news and news-gathering organizations, professional associations, universities, and journal and book publishers. Throughout the investigative and writing phases, our faithful companions included general, medical, and nursing dictionaries, as well as old and new texts on English composition and style. Dictionaries, in particular, proved to be invaluable resources; although they differed in the number of entries and methods of presenting information, many reported on the use of language.

In selecting content for the *Style Manual,* one of the most difficult and challenging aspects was deciding on appropriate descriptions and examples. This effort proved to be no easy task in light of the differing suggestions and contradictory views that appeared in the reference materials. In some instances, the differences seemed valid, indicating only a question of the writer's preference. Although we support flexibility in determining usage, we deliberately became arbitrary in certain situations. A case in point was the sequence of academic degrees and professional titles after a person's name. We strongly concurred with the experts from *The New York Times* and Associated Press, who recommended that academic degrees precede the professional designation. To illustrate, we believe that *Samantha Sinclair, PhD, RN,* represents the best or preferred form.

It is important to emphasize that this book covers American usage only, as reflected in the descriptions and spellings of words and phrases. Other nations have their own writing style preferences. A common error occurs in this country when writers spell *acknowledgment* with an extra "e" (*acknowledgement*). The latter choice may be the correct form in Great Britain or Canada, but it should not appear in U.S. writing. British spellings also differ in other ways, such as substituting an *s* for a *z* in words such as *organisation* (*organization*). An awareness of language conventions adopted by other lands is not only illuminating but beneficial for communicators as our world becomes smaller.

Although we share important principles of how to write well in this *Style Manual,* we also recognize that language is a fluid entity. It may distress the traditional grammarian to know that many of yesterday's taboos have disappeared, surrendering to popular expressions that border on jargon and slang. Fully aware of this pitfall, and with some discretion and good taste, we nevertheless have attempted to incorporate some of the more common changes and usage into this guide. You probably wonder what has accounted for this dramatic transformation of usage to a new acceptability. Yet, the inevitability of change should come as no surprise in an era of rapid technology development, the influence and spread of the Internet and e-mail, 24-hour cable news programs, and the imprecise language flowing from the lips of numerous talk show hosts. Furthermore, there is the phenomenal rise of political groups and their slogans teeming with misspellings and the mispronouncing of names and places.

As a motivator, the *Health Professionals Style Manual* will help you develop your own writing style—an elusive quality to describe, but one highly individualized because it reflects your personality and your *Weltanschauung* ("worldview"). No one said it better than E. B. White when he characterized style as the sound a writer's words make on paper. Like David Lambuth's earlier work on writing, Strunk and White's diminutive manual has more wisdom than many of the more expansive texts now available. Always keep both of these gems within reach!

In this book we have tried to cite the most useful material, hoping that there are no serious omissions. The content has undergone rigorous review by knowledgeable health professionals and editorial experts, and we invite you as representatives of the health care community and communicators in your respective fields to share with us your comments and suggestions for new areas of need. In the meantime, however, put *your* language to work!

Shirley H. Fondiller

Barbara J. Nerone

Foreword

Writing is easy. All you do is stare at a blank sheet of paper until drops of blood form on your forehead.

—Gene Fowler, novelist

I am not sure which (*who?*) is worse (*worst?*)—its (*it's?*) a toss-up (*jargon? colloquial?*). It is apparent (*to whom?*) that there is no consensus of opinion (*wordy?*) among (*between?*) editors. Is the writer that (*who?*) utilizes (*uses?*) cumbersome, pedantic, stilted, grammatically incorrect (*too many adjectives?*) language style as bad as the one who utilizes (*utilises if not a U.S.-based writer*) text-book (*no hyphen?*) perfect style and grammar (*grammer?*) but has no useful information? Well, perhaps, except for the fact that (*except that?*) I prefer people who pay attention to details and hate (*do I really?*) writers who think they are excellent writers but are not, yet correct everyone else's usage thus making it wrung (*too fast on spell check—should be wrong*) too (run-on sentence, flight of ideas, what *AM* I talking about?).

Okay, the above introduction to my foreword probably has impressed no one. The wording of the first paragraph was a device to make the point of how easy it is for writers to slip into *usage hell.* However, depending on who the reader of our writing is, not paying attention to style details or using an introductory paragraph like mine can lead to a D grade for grammar and composition on a school paper, outright rejection of a manuscript, instructions for a massive revision, and suggestions to get "editorial help." Poor language style also distracts readers; they wonder when the expression of the ideas is poor and sloppy, can the content be any better?

When presenting your ideas in a professional context, some colloquialism and style variation is inevitable, for example, using the word *which* to further describe something when *that* is the correct word, a dash when a semicolon is proper, *deceased* or *passed away* when *dead* or *died* better conveys intent, or having a few run-on sentences and splitting an infinitive. However, the purpose of writing is to effectively convey a message to an audience. Although a few style errors in your writing won't bother most readers, they will be noticed. The more you "get it right," the more readers will focus on your message (your content) and not poorly constructed sentences. Most readers will overlook style errors, but a certain number will always think less of you (and thus, your content) for not writing properly. Correct style is a matter of pleasing all your readers, not just some.

English grammar and composition, the backbone of all writing, is strongly influenced by how much attention we paid to our grade school instruction. That formative school content laid the foundation for how we write today. Since early school days, few of us have had more formal instruction in grammar and language usage. The expression of our ideas is more from habit than a deliberate thought process. Most of us do not *think* about the effort of writing—we just *know how to write* and feel our writing is certainly acceptable. Based on reading thousands of manuscripts, I know that writing well does not come naturally. I frequently read grammatically poor manuscripts, written by authors who are deans, vice presidents, and professors with master's and doctoral degrees. It is authors who understand there is always room for improvement (such as yourself because you are reading this book) who quickly learn to use grammar and composition techniques that do not interfere with or overshadow the message.

The *Health Professionals Style Manual* is a guide to improving your approach to good writing. As an example, the *Style Manual* can first be used as a review of style rules and then as a self-assessment resource to discover the rules you routinely break. This will immediately improve your composition style as self-awareness of your writing peculiarities increases. As with most language style guides, the content is prescriptive; it provides rules for writing. But remember, no set of rules covers every type of writing. Each vehicle used to convey your ideas—be it a journal, book, editorial, essay, letter to the editor, business report, thesis, or e-mail—has a different style and different format rules. The *Style Manual*'s authors advise you to spell out numbers from one to ten. The style for my journals requires use of Arabic numerals for all numbers starting with 1. By breaking a *Style Manual* "rule," you are following a "rule" in my guide.

When communicating your ideas, your goal is to learn what rules cannot be broken (the word *it* used as a possessive pronoun or adjective is always *its*—as in, its demise . . . *no apostrophe*) and what rules are just the preference (Arabic versus Roman numerals in tables) of someone (boss, teacher, editor) or some style resource. All style guides are just that—guides. The *Health Professionals Style Manual* and other resources are tools to make you as comfortable with the mechanics of writing as you are with your content. As your knowledge of linguistic style and expression improves, you can make more informed decisions about your writing style and composition. As you deliberately choose words and structures to best express your ideas, you give readers the gift of clear writing that more effectively conveys your content.

Suzanne P. Smith, EdD, RN, FAAN
Editor-in-Chief
Journal of Nursing Administration and *Nurse Educator*

Health Professionals
Style Manual

1

Style and Substance:
The Dynamic Duo

Your style as a writer is a way of expressing your distinctive personality in vocabulary, idiom, and sentence structure. How you use language is more than simply passing information from one person to another, but rather showing how you feel about the people you talk and write to and your relationship with them. Whether you are preparing a manuscript for publication, a paper to be presented at a conference, or a school assignment, your approach to the work will depend on the subject being explored and the intended audience. Always be mindful that consciously copying another person's style would be viewed as a form of plagiarism. A comparison of styles indicates the differences between accurate expression of thought and individuality, and the careless combining of words that may seem intelligible but reveal nothing more.

WRITING STYLES: FORMAL, INFORMAL, AND POPULAR

Writing styles are classified as formal, informal, and popular. Some overlap may occur between them, but they function under different conditions and accomplish different ends.

Formal Writing

Unlike our everyday speech, reports, essays, textbooks, and academic or technical works require more formally constructed language and tend to be impersonal and precise. In such cases, resist the temptation of interjecting colloquial phrases (conversational expressions). Also, avoid contractions and abbreviations in addition to a more specialized and complex vocabulary frequently used in the spoken word. One of the more common pitfalls to watch for is that formal language can become too wordy or convoluted. Scholarly writing may follow this pattern because it demands a complex structure with its own set of conventions and rules. You will be on safer ground by following the guidelines established by the editors of scholarly publications.

Informal Writing

Informal writing reflects the language spoken by people every day. It shows a relaxation of grammar, less concern with vocabulary, and shorter sentences without colons and semicolons. Colloquialisms, contractions, and writing in the first person are common. Informal writing generally appears in newspaper articles and columns.

Popular Writing

Writing in popular English may be characterized as "colorful," but it is usually inappropriate unless you are responding to a speech or a published source. Because it frequently borders on slang, you need to proceed with caution. Although enthusiasm may seem to compensate for imprecise meaning or a limited vocabulary in verbal expression, it will not work with the written word.

Here are some examples of changes in vocabulary in formal, informal, and popular writing:

Formal	Informal	Popular
comprehend	understand	get it
intoxicated	drunk	smashed
exhausted	tired	beat (or wiped out)
dejected	sad	bummed

2

From Principles to Practice: The Art of Effective Writing

At the outset, your outline or plan will lay out the direction as well as destination of what you intend to say. The reader needs to understand this as quickly as possible, or you will face the disappointment of losing your audience. In other words, grab that reader from the start!

PROTECT YOUR PARAGRAPHS

The major components of good writing include unity and transition of paragraphs, proper sentence structure, and the use of words that are clear, accurate, and vivid.

Paragraphs are designed as a group of more or less clearly related sentences that involve a subdivision of the thought. If you make them too long, they will be difficult to follow, or choppy if too short. Five to six well-developed, properly constructed sentences seem more than adequate for a paragraph. Keep in mind that the most emphatic positions in a piece of writing appear at the beginning and end of a paragraph.

To continue an idea from one sentence or paragraph to the next, a smooth transition or a bridge may be necessary to avoid creating a bump in crossing over. The term *transition* simply means "to change." A common way of performing transitions between sentences in a paragraph is to use connectives such as *however, therefore, on the other hand, meanwhile, at the same time, then,* and *afterward.*

> *She accompanied the technician into the room. Afterward, she called the lab to get the results of the blood test.*

Transitional words or phrases at the beginning of paragraphs form a logical link to the preceding paragraph. Some examples include *on the contrary, as a result, furthermore, therefore,* and *in addition to.* Transitional paragraphs aim to separate, summarize, compare or contrast, and emphasize.

STREAMLINE YOUR SENTENCES

As the unit of all logical thinking and writing, the sentence is primarily the setting up of an area of thought, known as the subject, and the saying of something about it, called the predicate. It represents the simplest form of making a complete and independent statement. Certain types of fragmentary writing are acceptable in modern usage but they must be applied judiciously, such as in the case of grouping certain words *without stating the verb.* The writer's intent is to show a simple perception: *Children bright and bubbly* or *a gust of wind.* These illustrations, referred to as impressionistic, give vitality to the writing but must be employed with circumspection.

Addressing the differences between simple, compound, and complex sentences will influence the presentation and clarity of style in structuring sentences. A simple sentence with a subject and predicate is a single statement of fact: *The administrator inspired staff loyalty.*

Compound sentences provide for a rudimentary grouping of statements but do not make it possible to distinguish clearly between the importance of connected statements. They tend to become stringy and lack cohesiveness: *The procedure was brief and the patient was discharged early.* On the other hand, complex sentences show the importance of one idea over another and emphasize the interrelation of ideas. They are desirable as well as essential in fostering accurate thinking: *Because of the brief procedure, the patient was discharged early.* In this example, the dominant idea becomes clear with the emphasis on the patient's discharge.

When developing your sentences, try to write them in crisp and concise language. Think of verbosity as the "curse" of the amateur and that a thought in its natural form is more understandable. Study the following examples to learn how to overcome three common faults: the clogged sentence, the overburdened sentence, and the too-complex sentence.

The Clogged Sentence

Clogged sentences lack precision and will clutter your writing with unnecessary words. To retain readers' interest, avoid clumsy language that obstructs the thought you wish to convey.

> Poor: *Lisa Martin, age 58, of 19 Briarwood Drive, who told the staff nurse that she had never been hospitalized and whose husband had died two months earlier in the same hospital, was reluctant to sign the consent form that would authorize her pending exploratory surgery.*

> Improved: *Lisa Martin was reluctant to sign the consent form for her pending exploratory surgery. The 58-year-old woman told the staff nurse that her husband had died in the same hospital two months earlier.*

The Overburdened Sentence

Similar to the clogged sentence, it is packed with ideas rather than facts.

> Poor: *Under the legislature's health plan for the past year, the proposed new amendment for health professional education now before the Health Education Committee, not only deals with funding for all types of nurse manpower but also for the creation of several new categories of health care technicians.*

> Improved: *The health professional amendment being proposed before Congressional committees not only deals with funding for nurses but also for new categories of health care technicians.*

The Too-Complex Sentence

This type of sentence resembles and sometimes combines clogged and overburdened sentences.

> Poor: *At the time of the critical nurse shortage during the late 1980s, and because of public concern over the crisis, especially in view of the fact that hospitals were closing units and turning away patients not only in the Northeast but all over the*

> *nation, the nursing profession mobilized its leadership to*
> *seek long-term solutions and not just immediate answers to*
> *this recurring problem in recruitment and retention.*

Improved: *Because of public concern with the nursing shortage of*
the late 1980s, the profession mobilized its leadership to
seek long-term solutions for a recurring problem. As a
result of the crisis, hospitals nationwide closed units and
turned away patients.

WATCH YOUR WORDS

Long ago, Alexander Pope described wordiness as follows:

> Words are like leaves, and where they most abound
> Much fruit of sense beneath is rarely found.
>
> —"An Essay on Criticism"

Scientific language is acceptable as well as necessary when writing to an audience of peers, who will understand such terms as *arteriotomy, palliation,* or *splenic sequestration.* At the same time, use these terms cautiously, and it may be better to define the terms at first mention. It is a "must" for a consumer audience.

To a large degree, proper sentence structure facilitates clarity of expression, while accuracy and vividness depend upon the words you use. Your selection of words must conform meaning to be conveyed to the reader. Words poorly chosen, misleading, and vague indicate that the writer has not been clear in getting the message across. The best rule for writing, as in speaking, is to use the *simplest* words. Pedantic prose will offend your audience and turn them off. Obscurity is not profundity!

As the bones and sinews of language, nouns and verbs represent the foundation of effective writing. Select them wisely with particular attention to appropriateness and accuracy. Voltaire was right on target when he declared that the "adjective is the enemy of the noun." Although often necessary to describe the writer's meaning and make it precise, adjectives can lessen the force of a sentence unless used sparingly. So, beware of overloading your sentences with adjectives for definiteness and adverbs for intensity. Whenever possible, select verbs that picture or imply action because they are busy doing or making something; for example, using *When Elizabeth reigned,* instead of *When Elizabeth was Queen,* makes your writing "swing." In your work, substitute *active verbs* because they add color and vitality. Substitute them also for such verbs as "to be, to have, to seem" and others of that overworked family.

A good tip essential for appropriate verbiage is to include the use of *specific* rather than *general* words, and *concrete* rather than *abstract* words. Specific words are more effective because they paint pictures of individual objects and reflect the writer's imagination and ability to observe carefully and express thoughts accurately.

General Words: *The nurse practitioner spoke frankly to the new patient.*

Specific Words: *Lauren Davis, the oncology nurse practitioner, explained the proposed treatment to Mrs. Connors, the new patient.*

When developing your ideas for a written work, try to avoid the use of abstract words, which appear vague and often pedantic. Concrete words, on the other hand, represent material that can be touched, seen, heard, and even smelled. They are more interesting, clear-cut, and move rapidly. The following example is reproduced from David Lambuth's classic work titled *The Golden Book on Writing* (1964):

Abstract Words: *Mortal existence is characterized by its transitoriousness and its fallacious appearance of importance.*

Concrete Words: *All the world's a stage, and all men and women merely players.*

In writing proper language, it is necessary to consider whether to indicate less than a 100 percent certainty. Expressing caution can be manifested by using the verbs and adverbs shown below:

Verbs	Adverbs
appears to	perhaps
seems to	possibly
tends to	probably
may	apparently
might	likely

The following illustrates definite and tentative (cautious) statements:

Definite: *The patient's health problem is exacerbated by her refusal to cooperate.*

Cautious: *The patient's health problem tends to be exacerbated by her refusal to cooperate.*

Definite: *The therapist was overwhelmed by the heavy client load.*

Cautious: *Perhaps the therapist would have been less overwhelmed with better scheduling of client appointments.*

WATCH FOR OVERUSED WORDS

The following words are frequently overused by writers. Although they are legitimate and at times may even seem more acceptable, an entire manuscript with too many of them sounds pretentious. Most of the alternative terms listed below are synonymous with the overworked word. Your selection will depend upon the use of the word in a sentence.

Keep in mind that these words can be eliminated by merely rephrasing the sentence. Your goal is to make your prose clear and easy to understand for the reader.

Overused Word	Alternative
abbreviate	shorten
accelerate	hasten
accomplish	carry out
accordingly	therefore
actuate	put into action, move
additional	added
aggregate	total
agitate	shake, stir, excite
alleviate	make easier
ameliorate	improve
anticipate	expect
antithesis	opposite

append	add
appropriate (adj.)	proper (adj.)
approximately	about
ascertain	find out
assimilate	absorb, digest
autonomous	independent, self-governing
beneficial	helpful
bilateral	two-sided
bottom line	final result, outcome
burnout	fatigue, exhaustion
circuitous	roundabout
coagulate	thicken
cognizant	aware
commence	begin
commodious	roomy
conception	thought, idea
conjecture	guess
consequently	so
considerable	much
contiguous	touching, near
criterion	rule, test
deficiency	lack
development	growth
deviate	turn aside
diminution	lessening
empower	enable, authorize
encounter	meet
facilitate	help
hence	so
indeed	in fact
indicate	show
ineffectual	useless
initiate	start, begin
innocuous	harmless
interface	communicate, interact
interrupt	hinder, stop
inundate	flood

isolate	apart
judicious	wise
liberate	free
likewise	and, also
lots, lots of	a great many
lucid	clear
luminous	bright
manifest	clear, plain
manufacture	make
meaningful	important, significant (if not over used)
minimal	smallest
mitigate	make mild, soften
modification	change
moreover	now, next
nebulous	hazy, vague
objective	aim, goal
oblique	slanting
observation	remark
observe	note
obsolete	out-of-date
occupy	take up, fill
operate	work, run
orifice	opening, hole
paradigm	pattern
parameter	boundary
partially	partly
penetrate	pierce
periphery	outer edge
present (verb)	give
problematical	doubtful
procure	get
purchase	buy
restructure	rebuild, reorganize, revamp
significant	important, striking, telling
super (slang)	wonderful, ideal, first-rate
terminated	died, ended, dismissed

thus	so
utilize	use

WATCH FOR EXTRA WORDS

Avoid	**Preferred**
a large number	many
a majority of	most
afford the opportunity	permit, allow
ahead of schedule	early
almost never	seldom
are of the opinion	believe
as of now	today
at this point in time	now
be kind enough	please
because of the fact that	because
comes in conflict with	conflicts
despite the fact that	although
due in large measure to	due largely to
during the time that	when
except for the fact that	except that
for the purpose of	for
for the reason that	because
for this reason	so
give enough encouragement to	encourage
give rise to	create
had occasion to be	was
in accordance with	according to
in advance of	before
in an impatient manner	impatiently
in favor of	for
in order to	to
in reference to	about
in the event that	if
in the nature of	like
in the near future	soon

in the neighborhood of	about
in the process of (preparing)	preparing
in view of the fact that	because
inasmuch as	because
it is often the case that	frequently
it is the intent	we (I) hope
of a confidential nature	confidentially
on account of	because
on the basis of	based on
on the grounds that	because
prior to	before
refer back to	refer to
take into consideration	consider
that is to say	in other words
to be sure	of course
until such time as	until, when
with regard to	regarding
with the result that	so that

3

Understanding Usage:
An Alphabetical Guide to
Specific Writing Tips and Pitfalls

A

<u>A, an.</u> Indefinite articles. Use <u>a</u> before words beginning with a consonant or consonant sound: *a nurse, a hospital, a procedure.* Use <u>an</u> before words beginning with a vowel sound: *an unknown origin, an inoperable tumor.* The use of <u>a</u> and <u>an</u> before abbreviations or numbers depends on the sound: *an NYU student, an IV, a two-step procedure, an eight-hour shift.*

Words beginning with <u>h</u>, when the initial <u>h</u> is not pronounced, are preceded by <u>an</u>.

> *Dr. Bond indicated that the therapy session would last an hour.*

A word with an <u>h</u> firmly emphasized in the first syllable is preceded by <u>a</u> and not <u>an</u>.

> *Her paper focused on a history of postanesthesia recovery rooms.*

> *Bette preferred a historical novel to an inflated autobiography.*

<u>Abbreviations, acronyms.</u> (See also Appendix A.) An <u>abbreviation</u> is a shortened form of a word or phrase used chiefly in writing to represent the complete form.

> *RN   Registered Nurse*

> *ANA   American Nurses Association*

> *MRI   magnetic resonance imaging*

Spell out a proper name or word the first time it is mentioned. Then use the abbreviation or acronym. Insert the abbreviation in parentheses following its first use.

> *Elliot had suffered a myocardial infarction in 2004. He hoped that it would be his only MI.*

> *The American Nurses Association (ANA) supports. . . . ANA also works toward . . .*

Be careful when using the same abbreviation for two different titles. For example, *AACN* is the abbreviation for both the *American Association of Critical Care Nurses* and the *American Association of Colleges of Nursing.* In such cases, spell out the proper name to avoid misunderstanding.

An acronym is a word formed with the first letter or letters of each of a series of words, such as *W.H.O.* for *World Health Organization* or *radar* for *radio detecting and ranging.* Do not be tempted to turn every committee name into an acronym. What may simplify a long name should not merely be used to have a clever acronym.

Do not use a period between the letters of an acronym except when they spell a word that might be misunderstood or when the acronym or abbreviation has another meaning. Examples are:

> *I.N.A.N.E.   International Academy of Nursing Editors*

> *W.H.O.   World Health Organization*

> *N.O.W.   National Organization for Women*

Academic degree. Use abbreviations such as MS or DNSc only after a full name and never after a last name appearing alone. The trend is to omit periods in abbreviations of academic degrees. Be consistent if you use them.

Academic degrees should precede professional titles. Some publications, however, reverse the order.

> *Eleanor Drake, PhD, RN* (more acceptable usage)

> *Eleanor Drake, RN, PhD*

The MD (doctor of medicine) and PhD (doctor of philosophy) are academic degrees. When both are stated, the order is determined by the first earned degree.

Jeremy Welby, MD, PhD (Dr. Welby earned his MD before the PhD.)

An honorary doctorate is not an earned degree and should not be listed as a credential after an individual's name. Also, do not refer to a person with an honorary degree as "Doctor," unless the individual also has an earned doctorate.

Although the BA, BS, and BSN are earned degrees, do not use them in a listing of credentials when followed by an advanced degree. The bachelor's degree is assumed.

Sara Scott, MA, RN

The above principle applies to the master's degree when a doctoral degree has been earned. An exception occurs with an earned degree in a different discipline, such as a PhD nurse with an MBA.

Lucie Anderson, MBA, PhD, RN

Although it is common practice in nursing to use the BS and BSN along with the RN in bylines and references, this usage rarely occurs in other disciplines. An English major or engineer, for example, never uses:

Mark Cummings, BA, director of sales, Columbia Computer Corporation

For the correct attribution when submitting a manuscript, check the format of the publication in which you wish to publish.

Academic and other titles.

a. *academic titles.* Capitalize when used before a person's name. Use lowercase, and set off with commas, after a name. Capitalize a school or college name when used alone or identified with a university, but lowercase academic departments or divisions.

Dean Claire Forbes

Claire Forbes, EdD, RN, dean, School of Nursing, Alpha University

George Martin, PhD, head, department of English, Ethan Allen College

Lesley Prince, DSc, professor, division of social sciences, Alpha University

Never address an individual as <u>Dr.</u> Claire Forbes, <u>EdD.</u> <u>Doctor</u> or <u>Dr.</u> applies to earned degrees, but its use before a name is commonly identified with medical doctors. Take care to identify a person's specialty if <u>Doctor</u> applies to other than a medical doctor.

> *Dr. Janet Van Franken, a registered nurse, writes . . .*

> *Janet Van Franken, DSc, RN* (preferred)

b. *professional titles.*

1. RN (Registered Nurse). Use after the surname except when other titles acknowledge the person as a registered nurse.
2. Certification designation (c). The certification symbol (c) appears after the academic degree. In recognizing certified nurses, eliminate the use of RN when the individual's degree is above the baccalaureate.

> *Sue Shekleton, DNSc, CNM* (certified nurse-midwife)

> *Jane Monroe, MA, CCRN* (certified critical care nurse)

3. FAAN (Fellow of the American Academy of Nursing). Place FAAN at the end of a person's complete title. It is unnecessary to put <u>RN</u> after the person's name because all members of the AAN are registered nurses. At the same time, if the audience does not associate FAAN with an RN, then include the latter title.

> *Margaret A. Lamberson, EdD, FAAN*

c. *titles in health care agencies or organizations.* Lowercase except for the name of a hospital, health agency, or organization.

> *Maybelle Crane, MA, CRNA, educational consultant, American Association of Nurse Anesthetists, Park Ridge, IL*

> *Amy Bottoms, MS, FAAN, clinical specialist in psychiatric nursing, Back Bay Mental Health Center, Boston*

> *Martin Johns, MS, assistant director, department of fiscal affairs, Johnson Memorial Medical Center, San Francisco*

Accept, except. Accept, a verb, means "to receive." Except, a preposition or conjunction, means "other than" or "but for."

> *Pearl was about to accept the beautiful bouquet when the embarrassed ballerina suddenly sneezed.*
>
> *The actor's performance pleased everyone except the impatient understudy.*

Also use except as a verb to mean "to leave out."

> *She was excepted from the new policy.*

Accreditation, approval. Not synonymous. State board approval is required to operate a medical or nursing school. Voluntary accreditation is desirable to ensure high standards.

Adapt, adopt. Use adapt to mean "to convert" and adopt to mean "to take as one's own."

> *We adapted the computer system to the peculiarities of our company.*
>
> *The staff reluctantly adopted the new computer system.*

Addendum. Singular noun. The plural is addenda, not addendums.

Advanced nursing practice. A term indicating nursing preparation at the master's degree and higher level. Generally refers to nurse practitioners, nurse anesthetists, nurse midwives, and clinical nurse specialists.

Adverbs. Adverbs describe verbs, adjectives, or other adverbs to add description and detail. Avoid the practice of creating adverbs by adding ly to an adjective and then combining it with a weak verb.

> Poor: *to discuss meaningfully*
>
> Improved: *to enlighten/to persuade/to explain*
>
> Poor: *to think conceptually*
>
> Improved: *to generate an idea/to conceive an idea*

Put adverbs normally between the elements of a compound verb.

> *We should clearly place more importance on the issue of ethical behavior.*

Do not split an infinitive with an adverb under most circumstances. See Verbals: split infinitive.

Adverse, averse. Adverse means "opposed to or unfavorable to." Averse means "unwilling to" or "reluctant to."

> *The committee's adverse remarks distressed the chairman.*
>
> *He was averse to undertaking the treatment.*

Advice, advise. Use advice as a noun, advise as a verb.

> *Hillary Marks gave her student valuable advice on career opportunities.*
>
> *The therapist advised her of the procedure's limitations.*

Adviser, advisor. Use either, but be consistent within the same work.

Affect, effect. As verbs, affect means "to influence or change," and effect means "to accomplish or cause."

> *Yo-yo dieting can severely affect your health.*
>
> *Good nutrition and an active lifestyle will effect a better sense of well-being.*

The noun, effect, means "result." The noun, affect, is a term reserved for use in psychological works.

> *One effect of IV drug use is the risk of getting HIV.*
>
> *The patient presented a disturbing affect that confirmed the therapist's diagnosis.*

Agenda. Singular. The plural, agendas, is rarely used.

> *No one knew the hidden agenda until the meeting concluded.*

Ages. Give the ages of people in numerals.

> *the 5-month-old boy; Margaret Smith, 43 years old*

Spell out the ages of inanimate objects or things nine and below, and use numerals above nine.

> *the 100-year-old facility, the five-year-old record*

An exception occurs when both categories appear in a sentence or paragraph discussion.

> *The one-hundred-year-old institute's twelve branches needed repair.*

Aggravate, annoy. Not interchangeable. Aggravate means "to make worse, more severe." Annoy means "to disturb or irritate."

> *Mr. Foote aggravated his back problem by lifting the computer.*
>
> *Do not annoy the patient with too many questions.*

Aid, aide. As a verb, aid means "to assist," as a noun, "assistance." Aide, a noun, means "an assistant."

> *Professor Smart aided her students in resolving the issue.*
>
> *The students appreciated Professor Smart's aid.*
>
> *The aide performed her tasks well.*

-al. Follow the practice of dropping the terminal al unless it changes the meaning.

> *Tanya's expertise was in the oncologic (not oncological) field.*
>
> *Lincoln's Gettysburg Address, although criticized by newspapers of the era, was considered a historic (not historical) event.*

A lot. Always written as two words meaning "much" or "many." Alot is not a word.

> *The social worker spent a lot of time contacting agencies.*

All ready, already. Used as a pronoun or adjective, all ready means "entirely prepared." Use already, an adverb, to mean "so soon" or "previously."

> *They were all ready to leave, but the discharge clerk kept them waiting.*

> *The operation was already delayed two hours.*

Allude, elude. Allude means "to make indirect reference"; elude means "to avoid or escape."

> *Explaining the new procedure, Roseanne alluded to a change in staffing.*

> *Tom skillfully eluded the instructor's demands.*

Alumnus, alumni/alumna, alumnae. An alumnus (alumni pl.) is "a man who has attended or graduated from an institute of higher learning."

An alumna (alumnae pl.) is the similar reference for a woman. Use alumni to refer to a group of men and women.

A.M., P.M., a.m., p.m. Upper or lowercase, with or without periods, it is your preference, but be consistent. Avoid redundancy such as *10:30 A.M. yesterday morning.* Often printed as small capitals: A.M. 6:00 A.M. is preferable to 6 A.M.

> *Surgery was scheduled for 8:00 A.M.* (not eight in the a.m.)

Among, between. Between applies to two people or things, and among to more than two: *between you and me, among the children.*

Amongst. Avoid use of this archaic form (from Middle English).

Ampersand (&). Symbol for "and." Use only in company names and abbreviations, such as AT&T, Smith & Wesson, but not in formal writing. An ampersand can be used in a reference before the name of the last author in a list of authors.

And etc. Because etc. means "and all the rest," the and in and etc. is unnecessary. Substitute and so on. See Latin derivatives.

And/or. Used primarily in legal and business writing. Avoid using in professional writing.

Anxious, eager, angst. Anxious, an adjective, usually means "nervous" or "worried," describing negative feelings. Eager, an adjective, means "enthusiastically anticipating," describing positive feelings. Angst, a noun, shows feelings of "anxiety, apprehension, or insecurity."

> *He was anxious about his medical report.*
>
> *They were anxious about the imminent birth of Murphy's baby.*
>
> *She was eager to sign the contract for her first book.*
>
> *Mark's wife awaited word of his medical condition filled with angst.*

Anyone, any one, anybody, any body. Anyone and anybody are pronouns. Any body is a noun modified by "any." Any one is a pronoun or adjective modified by "any."

> *Anyone can volunteer for the night shift.*
>
> *Will anybody help me with this task?*
>
> *I have more talent than any one person in this department.*

Anyplace. Avoid this informal expression meaning "anywhere."

Anyway, anywhere. Use anyway, anywhere, not anyways or anywheres.

Apostrophe. Apostrophes are used to:

- form the possessive of nouns not ending in s.

  the school's dean, the patient's prescription

- form the possessive of plural nouns ending in s. Use the apostrophe only; do not add an s.

  nurses' notes, doctors' rounds

- form the possessive of singular nouns ending in s or s sounds. Use either the apostrophe alone or 's.

  Burns' poetry, Burns's poetry

- An exception is the omission of the apostrophe in the proper names of most state and district nurses associations. This is consistent with the style of the American Nurses Association, as in the *Colorado Nurses Association.*

- form plurals of letters. Use 's if needed for clarity.

  13 i's, ABCs, CEOs, RNs

- indicate the omission of one or more letters or numerals.

  the 'gator, '99

- form the plural of numerals. The more generally accepted style is to omit the apostrophe.

  1950s, size 10s, the '60s

Appendix. Supplementary material usually attached at the end of a piece of writing. Plural: appendixes or appendices. Appendix is synonymous with addendum.

Appraise, apprize, apprise. Use appraise or apprize to mean "to evaluate." Use apprise for "to inform."

> *The autograph expert appraised* (or *apprized*) *the Nightingale letters but did not disclose their value.*
>
> *They apprised the tour leader of the hazardous driving conditions.*

Apt, likely, liable. These three adjectives have subtle differences. Apt means "well adapted"; likely means "probably, believable"; and liable means "legally obligated, responsible."

> *He made an apt choice.*
>
> *It was a likely story.*
>
> *She admitted being liable for her actions.*

Armed services, armed forces. Lowercase unless using the proper name of a specific branch of the military, such as *U.S. Army Nurse Corps.*

As, because, since. These three conjunctions have slight differences. Use as to convey a specific time instead of while or when. Because and since are interchangeable, showing cause and effect.

> *As the nurse prepared his medication, the patient watched her carefully.*
>
> *Because (since) the student's finances were limited, he bought used textbooks.*

As, like. As, a conjunction or preposition, is often confused with the preposition like. As means "similar" or "similarly to." The preposition like shows approximation or means the manner of, or having the same characteristics.

> *The students used the same equipment on one unit as they did earlier in the classroom.*
>
> *You can get your degree as I did.*
>
> *If he dresses like a physician, people may think he is one.*
>
> *Anita performed like a veteran and earned her Supervisor's respect.*
>
> *She fought like a terrier with a bone to have her opinion recognized.*
>
> *You can go to a university like the one suggested by your counselor.*

Like is never an adverb, although such usage has overwhelmed modern speech.

Assistance, assistants. Use assistance to mean "support or help." Assistants means "helpers."

> *Her client's assistance with the test hastened the results.*
>
> *He had openings for two assistants on the project.*

Assistant, associate. Use assistant for a "helper," associate for a "fellow worker" or "partner."

My assistant will show you the way.

My associate will prepare a draft of the budget.

In academia, an associate professor ranks below a full professor but above an assistant professor. Never abbreviate either term. Capitalize only when part of a formal title before a name.

Assistant Dean Margaret Clinton

Associate of arts, associate of science. Always use the full title when referring to the degree, usually earned from a junior or community college. *ADN* commonly refers to an associate degree in nursing.

Association. Capitalize the word when part of an organization's name, as in *American Association of Colleges of Nursing.* Otherwise, lowercase it.

Assure, ensure, insure. All verbs. Assure means "to promise" and refers to persons. Ensure and insure mean "to make certain," but the latter is preferred in legal and financial writing and usually implies formal protective measures.

I can assure you that the protocol will be followed.

Her hospitalization ensured proper care.

It is difficult to insure yourself against some natural disasters.

At large. Hyphenate only when used as an adjective.

She was elected as a delegate at large.

The delegate-at-large elections were held Saturday.

Author. In the narrative of an article with a byline, use a pronoun to express the author's point of view rather than writing "the author believes."

In my view . . . Rather than *In this author's view* . . .

I believe . . . Rather than *The author believes* . . .

Avoid using "to author" as a transitive verb.

Poor: *Jennifer Penn authored an excellent article on managed care.*

Improved: *Jennifer Penn was the author of an excellent article on managed care.*

Avant-garde. Always hyphenate.

Awful, awfully. Avoid in formal writing. Substitute a word that closely matches the intended meaning.

Poor: *Ms. Sanger had an awful delivery.*

Improved: *Ms. Sanger had a difficult delivery.*

A while, awhile. Use awhile, an adverb, as one word. Use a while (two words), a noun phrase, after a preposition.

The dean decided to wait awhile for the evaluations.

I will complete my introductory courses in a while.

B

Baby girl (or boy). A redundant phrase, as in *She delivered a baby girl.* No one is born fully grown.

She delivered a six-pound girl.

She delivered a six-pound daughter.

Baccalaureate. Means a "bachelor's degree." The term baccalaureate degree is redundant, although commonly used in education.

He earned his baccalaureate with honors.

Bachelor of arts, bachelor of science. Lowercase. Use BA or BS or bachelor's degree. BSN is the abbreviation for a bachelor of science degree in nursing. Always use an apostrophe in bachelor's or master's degree. It is acceptable to say bachelor's without the word degree.

Back of, in back of. Behind is a more acceptable choice.

> *He was behind the podium when the president approached the dais.*

Bad, badly. Bad is an adjective, badly an adverb.

> *He did a bad job on the report.*
>
> *He did badly on the entrance examination.*

Because of, due to. Use *because of*, a preposition, to mean "by reason of" or "on account of." Due to is unacceptable as a preposition meaning "because of." Use due to only after a form of the verb "to be" in formal writing.

> *Her irritable behavior was due to a lack of sleep.*
>
> *Because of* (not *due to*) *the patient's high fever, the surgery was postponed.*

Before, prior to. Prior to is used most frequently in a legal sense; before is used in almost all other cases.

> *Prior to rendering an opinion, Judge Eastwood requested a psychiatric evaluation of the felon.*
>
> *Before starting an infusion, the nurse checked her patient's oral intake.*

Being as/being that. Preference in formal writing is to use "since" or "because" rather than being as or being that.

> Poor: *Being as you asked, I'll be happy to help out.*
>
> Improved: *Since you asked, I will be happy to help out.*

Beside, besides. Beside, a preposition, means "next to." Besides, an adverb, means "in addition to."

Her colleagues stood beside her during the award ceremony.

Besides Ms. Hill, other people shared the organization's convictions.

<u>Besides</u> can also be a preposition meaning "in addition to" or "except."

There was no one in the OR suite besides the surgeon, the nurse, and the technician.

<u>Biannual, semiannual, biennial.</u> <u>Biannual</u> and <u>semiannual</u> are synonymous terms meaning twice a year; <u>biennial</u> means every two years.

He recommended a biannual checkup.

ANA has biennial conventions.

<u>Bias, prejudice.</u> <u>Bias</u> and <u>prejudice</u> both reflect a preconceived opinion, bent, or tendency, especially a sometime unreasoned judgment in favor or against a point of view. Prejudice generally shows unfavorable feelings.

Marta's bias was obvious in her voting record on the board.

Prejudice against businesswomen in management led to the expression "hitting the glass ceiling."

<u>Bimonthly, semimonthly.</u> <u>Bimonthly</u> means "every two months"; <u>semimonthly</u> is "twice a month." To avoid confusion, use <u>every two months</u> or <u>twice a month</u>.

<u>Black.</u> Lowercase. The term <u>African American</u> is preferred.

Poor: *black Americans, the black experience*

Improved: *African Americans, the African American experience*

<u>Blame on.</u> Avoid this term.

Poor: *His hospitalization was blamed on his forgetting to take the medicine.*

Improved: *They blamed his refusal to take his medicine for causing his hospitalization.*

Board of directors, board of trustees, governing board. Always lowercase except when used with the name of the organization.

The board of directors voted to suspend debate.

He was elected to the AHA Board of Trustees.

Buzzword. A word used by members of a particular discipline or profession. Usually a technical or important-sounding word used to impress laypersons. Avoid in formal writing.

C

Can, may. Use can to convey "ability" or "capacity" as well as "possibility." Use may to convey "permission."

She can run a successful business and still be a good wife and mother.

May I go to the workshop?

Capital, capitol. Lowercase when referring to capital, the city or town that is the seat of government. Uppercase when Capitol refers to a specific national or state building.

The nutritionists met with their representatives in the state capital.

The nutritionists lobbied their legislators at the State Capitol.

Capitalization. In general, limit capitalization to proper nouns.

a. *organizations.* Capitalize only when the official name of the entire organization, body, or group is given.

University of Minnesota School of Nursing, the school of nursing

the Board of Review for Baccalaureate and Higher Degree Programs, the board of review

the NLN Board of Directors, the board of directors, the board

Exception: Use <u>the League</u> when referring to the National League for Nursing. Refer to a constituent league as <u>the league</u>.

b. *titles.* Capitalize only in lists or when the title precedes the name.

> *Dean Donna Sharpe Donna Sharpe, dean of the school*
>
> *Executive Director David A. Bean, David A. Bean, executive director*

c. *courses, workshops.* Capitalize specific courses or workshops. No quotes. Lowercase the names of subjects.

> | | |
> |---|---|
> | *Ethical/Legal Aspects of Nursing* | *a course on ethics in nursing* |
> | *Chemistry 102* | *chemistry* |
> | *A conference on Patterns in Specialization: Challenge to the Curriculum* | *a conference on specialization in nursing* |

d. *acts, amendments, bills, laws.* Capitalize acts and laws when referring to their full title or the title by which they are commonly known, such as the *Ohio Nursing Practice Act.* Use lowercase if the act appears alone or in a general explanation.

> *The nursing practice act was one of many such examples.*

Lowercase the names of bills and amendments except when identified with the name of a sponsor, which is capitalized: *the Bradley bill.*

<u>*Caregiver, caretaker.*</u> Use <u>caregiver</u> in lieu of <u>caretaker</u> when referring to a person involved in the health care of an individual. <u>Caretaker</u> generally describes a person employed to take care of property.

<u>*Catalog, catalogue.*</u> <u>Catalog</u> is the preferred spelling, but be consistent.

<u>*Celsius.*</u> Named after the person who invented the centigrade system. Commonly used in scientific writing: *46 degrees Celsius* or *40° C.*

Center on, center around. Experts disagree about the appropriateness of either term in formal writing. Revolve around is often suggested as an alternative, and the prepositions at, in, and on are acceptable with center when you mean gathering or collection around an idea.

Poor: *His argument centered around his conviction that . . .*

Improved: *His argument revolved around his conviction that . . .*

His argument centered on his conviction that . . .

Chair, chairperson. Chairperson is the preferred alternative to chairman or chairwoman, particularly in academia and government. Use the term chair for either gender. Capitalize only when used as a formal title before a name.

Chairperson Marguerite Lopez called the meeting to order.

The chair called the meeting to order.

Check up, checkup. Use check up as verb, checkup as a noun.

Monica's anxiety delayed her checkup.

The new pharmacist decided to check up on the narcotics supply.

Cities and states. Capitalize names of cities and towns. Do not capitalize the word city unless it is part of the official name, such as *Kansas City*. Otherwise, lowercase, such as *the city of Boston*.

Unless a mailing address is given, the name of the state should follow the city except in the case of major cities, such as *Atlanta, Boston, Chicago, Los Angeles,* and *New York,* or if the state is obvious, such as *Iowa City.*

Spell out in full the name of a state when it stands alone, but abbreviate it when it follows the name of a city. Use the U.S. Postal Service abbreviations for state names.

Ohio   Columbus, OH; Oregon   Portland, OR

Spell out the name of a state when it follows the name of a county.

Montgomery County, Pennsylvania

Cook County, Illinois

Do not repeat the name of a state when it is included in the name of an institution or organization.

University of Minnesota, Minneapolis

Arkansas Department of Health, Little Rock

In all but major foreign cities, follow the name of the city with the full name of the country.

Amsterdam, London, Paris, Tokyo, New Delhi

Castlecomer, Ireland; Limoges, France

Enclose the abbreviation of a state in parenthesis when identifying the name of a hospital or health agency.

Coral Gables (FL) Memorial Medical Center

Clinical ladder. In nursing, this term refers to a system of recognition and reward to nurses meeting special criteria at different levels of practice. Also describes progress of the nurse advancing from one level or step to another.

Clinical nurse specialist. Refers to a registered nurse prepared at the master's degree level or higher in a clinical nursing specialty.

Collective nouns. Nouns such as committee, staff, team refer to a singular unit or group of individuals and are called collective nouns. Such nouns take a singular verb when they refer to the collection as a whole.

The staff was united on this project. (a unit)

The committee is meeting tomorrow. (a group)

A collective noun takes a plural verb when it refers to the members of the group as individuals.

The staff are always arguing among themselves. (individuals)

The committee are arriving for the meeting. (individuals)

Collective nouns normally taking singular verbs include:

Association
Board
Commission
Corporation
Cabinet
Committee
Commission
Government
Majority
Percent
Series
Council
Assembly
Audience
Class
Company
Couple
Family
Press
Half
Jury
Minority
Group
Information
Part (of)
Politics
Statistics
Crowd
Firm
Pair
Public
Staff

Collective nouns taking plural verbs include:

Assets
Headquarters
Proceeds
Scissors
Wages
Earnings
Means
Winnings
Odds
Premises
Savings
Series
Tactics
Wages

Some plural nouns, however, such as *measles, blues, mumps,* and *economics,* usually take a singular verb. Although the number is usually singular, the phrase, a number, is almost always plural.

A number of choices are available.

The number of choices is limited.

Colon. Marks the beginning of a phrase or sentence. Also used to introduce an important quote or a series. Capitalize the first word after a colon if a complete sentence follows.

His therapy served a purpose: It helped to build up his confidence.

His therapy could be described this way: effective, timely, and expensive.

Comma. Punctuation mark used to separate elements in a series, and generally before a conjunction. Often overused.

The top candidates were Joan, Jill, and Jessica.

Avoid the common error of inserting a comma to separate two or more verbs having the same subject.

> Poor: *The nurse took the chart, and recorded the patient's vital signs.*

> Improved: *The nurse took the chart and recorded the patient's vital signs.*

Use a comma to set off clauses that are <u>not essential</u> to the meaning of the sentence.

> *Her CPR course, which was scheduled for Tuesday, was canceled.*

Do not use a comma to set off clauses that <u>are essential</u> to the meaning of the sentence.

> *The man who was bald and limping was the chief suspect.*

<u>*Committee, commission.*</u> See <u>Collective nouns.</u> Capitalize only when part of a proper name. Do not abbreviate.

> *The commission issued a visionary report.*

> *The committee believes that its recommendations are sound.*

<u>*Company, companies.*</u> Capitalize only when part of a proper name, such as the *American Journal of Nursing Company.*

<u>*Compare to, with.*</u> Use <u>compare to</u> when the sense is "to consider or describe resemblances between unlike things." Use <u>compare with</u> to show similarities or differences between two like things.

> *The committee compared the woman's report of the incident to a soap opera script.*

> *You could never compare his level of commitment with hers.*

> *The primary physician compared his innovative treatment with the traditional approach of his predecessor.*

<u>*Compass points.*</u>

a. <u>*east (west, north, south).*</u> Capitalize when referring to a geographic region of the country or part of a proper name. Lowercase when you mean a point on a compass.

He left the South to find his fame and fortune on Broadway.

Proceed west on Route 138 for 5 miles.

Nursing in the Midwest is quite advanced.

She attended a baccalaureate program on the East Coast.

North Carolina, West Virginia

b. *eastern (western, northern, southern)*. Capitalize when referring to a geographic area of the country.

Bill has a Southern accent.

Milly is a Northerner.

Lowercase to designate compass points of a section of a state or city.

western New Hampshire

southern Dallas

It is acceptable, however, to capitalize widely known compass points such as *Southern California* or *Lower East Side of New York*. If in doubt, use lowercase.

Complement, compliment. Noun or verb. Complement means "that which completes or makes perfect." A compliment is an "expression of praise."

The support of the family complemented the patient's treatment.

The physical therapist complimented the elderly woman on her progress.

Complementary, complimentary. Use complementary to mean "serving as a complement, completing"; use complimentary to mean "given as an act of courtesy" and, in some cases, "free."

The efforts of the health care team showed a complementary relationship.

She received a complimentary book for her efforts.

Compose, comprise, consist of, constitute. These commonly misused words have subtle differences.

- Compose: "to create or put together"
- Comprise: "to contain; to include for all to embrace"
- Consist of: "to be made up of"
- Constitute: "to make up or form"

The nutritionist composed a 24-hour instruction plan.

Two nurses, a physician, and an administrator comprised the committee.

Seventy percent of the board constitutes a quorum.

His breakfast consisted of cereal, milk, and fruit.

Conference, congress, convention. Capitalize when part of a proper noun or as a title of an event. Otherwise, lowercase.

The National Council of State Boards of Nursing Conference featured an outstanding program.

The ICN Congress drew thousands of international participants.

APHA held its recent convention in Washington, DC.

Conform to, conform with. Use conform to when the idea of obedience is implied, such as *He demanded that all reports conform to one style.*

Conformity with is used to imply agreement: *His action plan was in conformity with the board's mission statement.*

Congressman, congresswoman. Capitalize only when used with a proper name. For example, refer to a member of the House as *Representative Barbara Sparks;* thereafter, refer to the individual as *the congresswoman.*

Connote, denote. Connote means "to suggest or imply something beyond the explicit meaning." Denote means "to be explicit about the meaning."

To some nurses, the concept of graduate education for certification connotes a threat.

To others, certification denotes the appropriate mechanism for fostering higher standards in nursing.

Continual, continuous. Use <u>continual</u> to mean "repeated often" or "intermittent," and <u>continuous</u> to mean "uninterrupted, without stopping."

Her continual habit of forgetting to take the medicine frustrated her family.

The award recognized the association's continuous support of health care reform.

Contractions. <u>Contractions</u> are words formed by the omission of a letter, such as *it's* (for <u>it is</u>). Although acceptable in informal writing, they should not be used in formal writing.

Frequently used contractions include:

it's	it is
they're	they are
aren't	are not
don't	do not
doesn't	does not

Contrast to, contrast with. Use <u>contrast to</u> when referring to something "opposite," and <u>contrast with</u> to mean "different."

Her reaction to the diagnosis was in contrast to her husband's response.

The contrast with her staff's opinion appeared obvious to everyone but the nurse manager.

Council, counsel. Use <u>council</u>, a noun, to mean "a group of advisers." Use <u>counsel</u>, a verb, to mean "to give advice." As a noun, <u>counsel</u> means "advice given."

The President's Council meets bimonthly.

They counsel recovering alcoholics.

She followed the counsel of the chief financial officer.

Credible, creditable, credulous. Use <u>credible</u> to mean "believable" and <u>creditable</u> to mean "worthy." A <u>credulous</u> person is "gullible."

The report was complicated but appeared credible to the nurse executives.

In substituting for her colleague, Ms. Jones gave a creditable performance.

The credulous student concurred with the instructor's analysis.

Criteria, criterion. Use <u>criteria,</u> the plural of <u>criterion</u>, to mean "standards for judgment."

Of all the criteria for selecting the candidate, character was considered the most important criterion.

Current, present. Synonymous terms meaning "belonging in the present" or "generally accepted."

The past results were low, whereas the current figures showed improvement.

In many cases, use of either word is unnecessary.

Poor :   *The current president of Sigma Theta Tau International will speak.*

Improved: *The president of Sigma Theta Tau International will speak.*

Currently, presently. Synonymous adverbs. It is more acceptable, however, to use <u>presently</u> to mean "shortly, soon, or now."

The discharge planner is (currently) unavailable but will be here presently.

Curriculum. The preferred plural is <u>curricula</u>, although <u>curriculums</u> may be used.

Cutoff, cut off. Use the noun <u>cutoff</u> to mean a "termination point." Do not use as an adjective. <u>Cut off</u>, a verb, means "to interrupt or sever."

> *The cutoff for the application is February 1.*

> *The moderator cut off the panelist who spoke too long.*

D

Dash. Punctuation mark showing a break in thought in a sentence, or emphasizing an appositive, or setting off parenthetical phrases.

> *In addition to the large group meetings, there were seven smaller breakout sessions—led by trained facilitators—whereby each participant remained with the same group and leader throughout the conference.*

Avoid using the dash when a comma will suffice.

> Poor: *These three elements—character, compassion, and credentials—combine to produce a qualified candidate.*

> Improved: *These three elements, character, compassion, and credentials, combine to produce a qualified candidate.*

Datum, data. Use <u>data</u> as the plural of <u>datum</u> in formal writing. <u>Data</u> can be used as both a plural noun taking a plural verb and plural modifiers and as a collective noun taking a singular verb and singular modifiers. Both uses are standard, but the plural usage is more common in print. In lieu of <u>datum</u>, use <u>fact</u> or <u>figure</u>.

> *The data is carefully recorded into the computer.*

> *The data are valid.*

Days of the week. Always capitalize. Abbreviate in a manuscript only when used in a tabular format.

Diagnosis, prognosis. Diagnosis identifies a disease through examination; prognosis predicts the disease outcome.

Dietitian, nutritionist. A dietitian is a person specializing in the study of nutrition as it relates to health. A nutritionist is an expert in the study of foods in general.

> *The hospital dietitian is responsible for planning patients' meals.*
>
> *She attributed her weight loss and energy to the nutritionist's instruction.*

Differ from, differ with. Use differ from to demonstrate items that are "unlike." Differ with shows disagreement.

> *The therapists differ from each other on the course of treatment.*
>
> *I differ with her political views.*

Different from, different than. Generally use different from except when a clause follows. Use different than when different from would sound awkward.

> *The protocols this year are different from those followed last year.*
>
> *It's a different protocol than it was 15 years ago.* (Different from would sound awkward in this construction.)

Dilemma. Watch the spelling and meaning of this word. A dilemma is not just a problem, but one that involves a choice between two undesirable alternatives.

> *The dilemma facing her was either to report the mistake or to respect her best friend's confidence.*

Discreet, discrete. Use discreet to mean "tactful," and discrete for "separate."

> *She offered a discreet comment about the controversy.*
>
> *They discussed the discrete elements of the plan.*

Disease entities. Do not capitalize a disease entity unless used with a proper noun: *cancer, asthma, coronary disease, Bright's disease, Hodgkins's disease, Alzheimer's disease.* Lowercase for procedures such as *cesarean* (or *cesarian*) *section.*

Disinterested, uninterested. Use disinterested to mean "unbiased or impartial," uninterested for "bored or lacking interest."

> *Most staff nurses were disinterested in the outcome of the dispute.*
>
> *The technician was uninterested in her explanation of the problem.*

Doctorate. A noun synonymous with doctoral degree. Do not use as an adjective.

> Poor: *Jerry was proud of earning his doctorate degree.*
>
> Improved: *Jerry was proud of earning his doctoral degree* (or *his doctorate*).

Documentation. See Referencing, Appendix F.

Domestic violence. Use instead of family abuse.

Dose, dosage. Use dosage to mean "a prescribed amount of a therapeutic agent." Dose, an abbreviation, is an "agent taken at one time or at stated intervals."

> *The dosage prescribed for Mr. Payne's headache was ineffective.*
>
> *The primary nurse gave the patient his 10 o'clock dose of pain medication.*

Double negatives. Always unacceptable.

> Poor: *The unit clerk did not have nothing to do on her personal day.*
>
> Improved: *The unit clerk did not have anything to do on her personal day.*

Doubt that, doubt whether, doubt if. Use <u>doubt that</u> to express conviction, <u>doubt whether</u> and <u>doubt if</u> to show uncertainty.

> *I doubt that she intended to hurt his feelings.*
>
> *I doubt whether (if) the board understood the ramifications of its decision.*

E

e-mail. Always hyphenate and lowercase.

Each, every. Use <u>each</u> or <u>every</u> in place of phrases such as <u>each and every</u>.

> *Each of us agreed with the diagnosis.*
>
> *Every one of the patients was awake and hungry.*

When used as a pronoun, <u>each</u> takes a singular verb.

> *Each was well educated for the task at hand.*

When <u>each</u> follows a plural subject, the verb agrees with the subject.

> *The patients each have separate rooms.*

Editor in chief. The preferred style is not to hyphenate; however, you should follow the style of the journal or the individual's title as indicated in correspondence.

E.g. See <u>Latin derivatives</u>.

Elaborate. Avoid adding the word "on," such as *elaborate on his position.*

-elect. Always hyphenate words formed with –elect, such as *president-elect, chairperson-elect.*

Ellipses. <u>Ellipses</u> marks (. . .) appear in threes and fours. Three dots represent words omitted from within or at the beginning of a sentence. Four dots (actually a period linked to three dots) show that words have been omitted at the end of a sentence or that sentences have been omitted from a paragraph.

Emigrate, immigrate. A person emigrates from a country. A person immigrates to a country to settle there.

> *Anna emigrated from Ukraine.*
>
> *He immigrated to the United States as a child.*

Eminent, imminent. Use eminent to mean "distinguished," imminent to mean "something about to occur."

> *The eminent scientist keynoted the convention.*
>
> *The beginning of the convention processional was imminent.*

End run, end-run. Both the noun, end run, and the transitive verb, end-run, are acceptable in speech and everyday writing, but should not be used in formal writing.

Especially, particularly, specially. Especially and particularly are interchangeable. Specially means "for a specific reason."

> *I especially (particularly) enjoy the fringe benefits of my job.*
>
> *This style manual is specially designed for those in the health-care field.*

Essential clauses. Clauses are essential if they restrict the meaning. No comma is necessary.

> *Undergraduate students who have a 3.5 average are eligible for the dean's list.*
>
> *Deadlines that are not met age editors prematurely.*

Et al. See Latin derivatives.

Et cetera. See Latin derivatives.

Ever so often, every so often. Ever so often should be used when you mean something happens very often. Every so often means something happens only occasionally.

She was late for the team meeting ever so often.

Every so often Charles attended a CE program to the delight of his supervisor.

Everyone, everybody. Synonymous as pronouns that take a singular verb.

Ex-. In formal writing use <u>former</u>, rather an <u>ex-</u>.

The decline in cigarette smoking among American adults has resulted in many healthier former smokers.

Exam/examination. Use <u>examination</u> in formal writing and <u>exam</u> for everyday communication.

Exclamation (!). Reserve this punctuation mark for true exclamations or commands. Do not use merely to emphasize a simple statement.

It was an exciting conference.

What an exciting conference!

Expired. Use <u>died</u> rather than <u>expired</u> or <u>passed away</u>.

Poor: *Mr. Welles collapsed on the steps and expired within minutes.*

Improved: *Mr. Welles collapsed on the steps and died within minutes.*

Explicit, implicit. Use <u>explicit</u> to mean "clearly defined," <u>implicit</u> to mean "implied" or "understood."

We have an implicit understanding that the children may not watch movies containing explicit sex.

F

Farther, further. Use <u>farther</u>, an adverb, to show physical space; use <u>further</u> as an adjective or adverb to indicate "for an additional time," "in a greater amount," or in relation to abstract ideas.

The ambulance was farther from the hospital than she thought.

She did not wish to discuss the issue further.

Needing further consultation, the attending physician called in his colleagues.

Nothing is further from the truth.

Use <u>further</u> as a verb to mean "to advance."

She needed to further her education to get the promotion she wanted.

<u>*Federal.*</u> Capitalize for corporate or governmental bodies that use the word as part of their formal names: *the Federal Trade Commission, Federal Express.* More common practice is to lowercase when used as an adjective synonymous with the United States, such as *federal judge, federal agents, federal grants,* and so on.

<u>*Feminist.*</u> Describes a person of either sex whose beliefs and behavior are based on social, economic, and political equality of the sexes.

<u>*Fewer, less.*</u> Use <u>fewer</u> when referring to a number or group of individual persons or items. <u>Less</u> refers to quantities of abstract or unnumbered entities. Both words imply comparison.

The medical school received fewer applications from men last year.

The medical center received less criticism than its board of directors expected.

<u>*Figurative language.*</u> Refers to words used nonliterally. The basis of <u>figurative language</u> is comparison or association of two ordinarily separate things or ideas. Become familiar with the following common figures of speech:

a. *metaphor.* An implied nonliteral comparison. Avoid using <u>like</u> or <u>as</u>, or other words implying a comparison. Examples of metaphors are:

Why then the world's mine oyster. . . . ("The Merry Wives of Windsor," William Shakespeare)

This is <u>the porcelain clay of humankind.</u> ("Don Sebastian," John Dryden)

> . . . *leave behind us footprints on the sands of time.* ("Psalm of Life,"
> Henry Wadsworth Longfellow)

Avoid trite metaphors such as *cradle of the deep* or *captain of my soul.*

b. *mixed metaphors.* Two or more dissimilar images presented in rapid succession. Avoid using.

> *The medical center fiscally solved a sea of problems when unexpected funding propelled it into the lap of luxury.*

c. *simile.* A nonliteral comparison of two things dissimilar in most respects but similar to each other. Usually introduced by "like" or "as." Use sparingly in your writing, if at all.

> *When he defected from the Party, he acted like a bird out of a cage.*

Avoid trite similes such as *soft as a kitten, happy as a lark, pretty as a picture, hard as nails,* and *nutty as a fruitcake* (slang).

Figuratively, literally. Use figuratively to mean "involving a figure of speech or emblematic." It implies a nonfactual statement. Literally means "actually."

> *Observing her first operation, the young student literally fainted at the open operating sight.*

> *The evaluations committee described her proposal figuratively as a fairy tale.*

First, firstly. First, second, and so on are preferred, although firstly, secondly, and so on are grammatically correct. Be consistent in the form used.

Flout/flaunt. Use flaunt to mean "to show off." Use flout to mean "to treat with contemptuous disregard."

> *He flouted convention when he flaunted his raise.*

Following, after. An adjective, following means "coming next in order." After, a preposition, means "behind in place or sequence."

Watch for the following protocol.

She spoke after the award luncheon. (Never use *following the luncheon.*)

Follow-through, follow-up. These words are normally used as nouns. Follow-up can also be an adjective. When used as verbs, the hyphen is eliminated.

His follow-through is very poor.

Let's follow up on his suggestions immediately.

Our follow-up procedures need to be amended.

Footnotes. See Referencing, Appendix F.

Foreword, forward. Use the noun foreword for an introductory section of a book. As a verb, forward means "to advance"; as an adjective, it means "ahead" or "front."

Ms. Joslin wrote an excellent foreword to the text on diabetes education.

Please move forward or we will miss the speaker.

The forward pass was the chief weapon in the quarterback's arsenal.

Formally, formerly. Use formally to mean "in a formal manner" and formerly to mean "previously."

The chairperson formally convened the curriculum committee.

She practiced formerly in a community health agency in Atlanta.

Former, latter. An adjective, former means "something that occurred earlier in time, or that which came before." As a noun, it means "the first of two items." Use latter to refer to the second of a pair.

Her former employer was his former wife.

When Jay had to choose between a salad and soup, he selected the former.

Johnny and Ed are being interviewed, but the latter may drop out of the running.

Full-time, full time/part-time, part time. Hyphenate when used as an adjective, but not as a noun or adverb.

She has a full-time job.

She works full time.

Fulsome. Adjective meaning "offensively lavish." It is not synonymous with profuse. The use of the term fulsome praise to mean "abundant" is ambiguous and might cause confusion. The use of abundant or full leaves no doubt of the meaning.

G

Gentleman, gentlemen/gentlelady, gentleladies. Man or men/woman or women is preferred.

Geriatric nursing, gerontological nursing. Geriatric nursing literally means "nursing care of the aged." Gerontological nursing means "nursing care of the aged with emphasis on health, rather than on illness." Despite the different shades of meaning, the terms are often used interchangeably as in geriatric nurse practitioner (or specialist) and gerontological nurse practitioner (or specialist).

Geriatrics, gerontology. Not interchangeable. Geriatrics is the branch of medicine that deals with the diagnosis and treatment of diseases and problems specific to the aged. Gerontology is the scientific study of the biological, psychological, and sociological phenomena associated with old age and aging.

Gerunds. See Verbals.

Girl. Do not use in reference to a woman or a young woman. College student is preferable to college girl.

Good, well. Good, an adjective, describes someone or something. Well, an adverb, describes action. When used with verbs such as "look," "to be," or "feel," well refers to a state of health.

> *She is a good physician, but a difficult patient.*
>
> *The staff on 2-Miller works well together.*
>
> *The project is going well.*
>
> *I feel well.*
>
> *She looks well after her illness.*

Got, gotten. As the past participle and the simple past tense of get, got is preferred to gotten, which is the colloquial past participle of get.

> *She finally got the message.* (past)
>
> *He did not mean to volunteer, but he got caught up in the enthusiasm of the event.*

Government. Lowercase. Never abbreviate.

> *the federal government, the state government, the U.S. government*

Governmental bodies. Use full names. Capitalize the full proper name of governmental agencies, department, and offices: *U.S. Department of Health and Human Services.* Lowercase further mention of the name, such as *the department.*

Graduate, graduated. Always use from with the verb graduate.

> Poor: *She graduated Teachers College, Columbia University.*
>
> Improved: *She graduated from Teachers College, Columbia University.*

Grass roots. Two words. When used as an adjective, hyphenate.

> *The grass-roots message required immediate action on a national insurance plan.*

When used as a noun, <u>grass roots</u> can take either a singular or plural verb.

> *The grass roots is (<u>are</u>) concerned about the economy.*

H

Health care. Two words, but observe exceptions in formal names such as the *Joint Commission on Accreditation of Healthcare Agencies*. Hyphenate sparingly when used as an adjective.

> *The health-care industry is flourishing.*
>
> *The nurses provide home health care.*

Healthful, healthy. Use <u>healthful</u> to mean "conducive to good health" and <u>healthy</u> to mean "possessing good health."

> *In addition to being healthy, the nutritionist recommended healthful foods to her clients.*

Help, help but. Avoid the phrase <u>help but</u>.

> Poor: *He couldn't help but admire her commitment.*
>
> Improved: *He couldn't help admiring her commitment.*

Historic, historical. A <u>historic</u> event is one that stands out in history. A <u>historical</u> event refers to any past occurrence.

> *The Visiting Nurses Service of New York's 100th anniversary in 1993 was a historic event.*
>
> *At the convention, the organization displayed many historical materials.*

Home care. Two words. Hyphenate sparingly when used as an adjective.

Homosexual, lesbian. Use these terms rather than <u>gay</u> in formal writing.

Hopefully. Hopefully is an adverb meaning "with hope." Avoid using hopefully in formal writing when you mean "it is hoped" or "I hope."

> Poor: *Hopefully, writers will master the use of the word "hopefully."*

> Improved: *I hope that writers will strive to master the use of the word "hopefully."*

However. According to most grammarians, it is not correct to begin a sentence with however.

> Poor: *The film received a favorable review. However, it did not meet the expectations of the audience.*

> Improved: *The film received a favorable review. It did not, however, meet the expectations of the audience.*

To avoid such binds, rework as a complex sentence.

> *Although the film received a favorable review, it did not meet the audience's expectations.*

Hubris. A noun meaning "exaggerated pride or self-confidence." Dangerously close to becoming jargon.

Human, humane. Do not be confused by these two adjectives. Humane means "compassionate," but human means "pertaining to the human race."

> *Her humane care was one reason for her popularity among patients.*

Hyphen. Follow these two principles when using a hyphen: First, never divide words of one syllable; second, hyphenate only between syllables.

Use a hyphen to avoid ambiguity when forming a single idea from two or more words.

> *Mayor Smart will confer with the city's small-business employers about the proposal.*

> *He re-covered the wound with a sterile dressing.*

Do not hyphenate an adverb ending in <u>ly</u> and a participle, such as *easily remembered dosages* or *slowly moving car.*

Use hyphens between two or more modifiers that express a single thought.

> *a full-time employee*
>
> *300-bed hospital*
>
> *anxiety-provoking situation*

I

I. Use of the pronoun <u>I</u> in a manuscript can be effective if it is not over-done. Check the style of the target publication. Former United Press International editor Roger Tatarian said: "There should be enough of it [I] to give the flavor of the letter to the folks at home, but not so much as to make the writer hog the center of the stage."

I.e. See <u>Latin</u> derivatives.

<u>*Idiom.*</u> An expression useful to a specific profession, group of people, or region in one country. <u>Idioms</u> are considered slang or near slang and should not be used in professional writing. Some examples include *get the upper hand, keep tabs on, gone to the dogs, strike a bargain.*

<u>*If, whether.*</u> Use <u>whether</u>, rather than <u>if</u>, to begin a subordinate clause when the clause puts forth a choice.

> *Charles did not know whether to stay until the end of the meeting or leave early.*

<u>*Impact.*</u> A noun or verb indicating "forceful contact."

> *The rock impacted the car and forced the driver to lose control.*

In formal writing, do not use <u>impact</u> as a verb to mean "having an effect on."

> Poor: *The decision impacted the association.*
>
> *His sexist attitude impacted on her decision to leave her job.*

Improved: *The decision had an impact on the association.*

His sexist attitude had an impact on her decision to leave her job.

Imply, infer. Not synonymous. Imply means "to suggest or to hint." Infer means "to conclude from evidence or to draw a conclusion." A speaker implies something, whereas the listener infers something from a speaker.

> *The lab report implies serious problems ahead.*

> *The results of the lab test led us to infer serious problems ahead.*

In, into. Use in to indicate a state or position. Into describes a movement to an interior location or condition.

> *He was suffering in his anguish.*

> *Throw the recyclables into the bin!*

Incredible, incredulous. Incredible means "unbelievable"; incredulous means "skeptical."

> *His explanation was incredible.*

> *The administrator tossed him an incredulous stare.*

Individual, person, party. Use individual when you want to stress unique-ness or when you are writing about a single human being.

> *What right does an individual have to challenge the ruling?*

Use person in other contexts, such as *most persons would agree with that.* Party refers to a group, such as *a party of five for dinner.*

Infinitive, split infinitive. See Verbals.

Ingenious, ingenuous, disingenuous. A confusing trio of similar-sounding words that differ in meaning.

Ingenious means "showing imagination."
Ingenuous means "innocent or lacking sophistication."
Disingenuous means "crafty, not straightforward."

The staff praised her ingenious solution to the problem.

The ingenuous newcomer captivated her classmates.

His disingenuous comments aroused suspicion.

Input. As a noun and a verb, input is a technical term to describe information entered into a computer or word processor. Input, a noun, also means "amount entered to achieve output," such as an *input of fuel*.

The statistician used her data as input for the computer.

She spent hours inputting the information into the new database.

In professional writing, avoid using input as a noun meaning "general information" when information or data will suffice.

Poor: *She received valuable input for her report.*

Improved: *She received valuable information (data) for her report.*

In-service. Hyphenate this adjective. Never convert the adjective in-service to a noun or verb.

Poor: *We will in-service the new staff next week.*

Improved: *We will begin the staff's in-service program next week.*

Introductory expressions. Set off by commas, such expressions include for example, namely, such as, and that is. If the break in continuity is minor, no comma is necessary. Use a semicolon or a dash for a major break.

The computer output, for example, was a daily printout on each patient.

The instructor postponed the assignment, namely the two essays.

Ipso facto. Means "by the fact itself."

> *A nurse's aide, ipso facto, cannot prescribe medication.*

Italics. Italicize or underline names of books, newspapers, and magazines. Use quotation marks around the titles of chapters, articles, lectures, or speech titles, television programs, movies, plays, poems, or song titles.

> *The Journal of Nursing Scholarship has a wide distribution.*
>
> *Most academics follow The Chronicle of Higher Education.*
>
> *The children repeatedly asked to watch the videotape of "Snow White and the Seven Dwarfs."*

In general, italics should be employed sparingly, but they can be used to add emphasis to a word in a quotation. In such a case, you would have to insert (after the italicized word) within brackets the phrase *italics added.*

Keep in mind that after a term or word has been used, the italics are not repeated. Also note that italics are to be avoided with certain abbreviations, foreign phrases, and Greek letters. Some examples include et al., vis-à-vis, per se, a priori, and ad lib.

It's, its. It's is a contraction meaning "it is." Its is the possessive form of the pronoun "it."

> *It's the unit's decision to determine its staff scheduling.*

-ize. See Verb usage: avoid converting nouns into verbs.

J

Jargon. A special language of a trade, profession, class, fellowship, or region of the country. Idioms fall within this category. Avoid "jargonitis" such as:

Give him some TLC.

Ground the patient.

Check the meds.

K

Kids. Skip such colloquial expressions in formal writing. Substitute children.

Kind, kinds. Use with the demonstrative pronouns this, that, these, and those: *this kind, these kinds, those kinds.*

Know-how. A trite expression that should be avoided in formal writing.

Kudos. Takes a singular verb. Avoid using kudo.

L

Lady, woman. Use woman, not lady, in professional writing.

Last, past. Use last to mean "most recent," past to mean "elapsed time or location."

> *Margo Preston was elected chairperson at the group's last convention.*
>
> *The smell of cotton candy evoked a memory of summers past.*

Latin derivatives. Avoid Latin derivatives in formal writing. Spell out the English translation; however, it is acceptable to use the abbreviation within parentheses. The most common examples are:

e.g. = *exempli grata* = for example. Use only if the illustration being offered is one of several examples.
et al. = *et alii* = and other people (acceptable in citations only).
etc. = *et cetera* = and other things (literal). And so on is preferable.
i.e. = *id est* = that is. Used to interpret a previous statement (in which case you probably should have said it more clearly the first time) or to present an exhaustive list of examples.

[sic] = *thus, this way.* Use in square brackets to show your reader that an oddity in spelling or usage is in the original and not your error.

viz. = *videlicet* = namely

Lay, lie. Lay means to place or put in a particular position. It always takes a direct object (transitive verb).

I lay	*We lay*
You lay	*You lay*
He/she/it lays	*They lay*

Laid is the past tense and past participle. Laying is the present participle.

She laid the dressing on the sterile area.

She is laying the report on the table.

Please lay your head on my shoulder.

Lie means a "state of reclining" and does not take a direct object (intransitive verb). Past tense is lay, part participle is lain, and the present participle is lying. Lie also means "making an untrue statement."

I lie	*We lie*
You lie	*You lie*
H/she/it lies	*They lie*

The patient lies quietly in her bed.

He had lain for a long time on the examining table.

She is lying on the unaffected side.

The report lay on the table.

He was terminated from the project because he lied consistently.

Lead, led. As a verb, lead means "to take or conduct." Led is the past tense of lead.

The aide agreed to lead the family into the waiting room.

She led the people through the new wing.

Leave, let. Interchangeable only when followed by alone. Otherwise, let means "to allow" and leave means "to depart."

Leave (let) the report alone.

Let the patient see the report.

Legislative titles. Capitalize titles used with proper names. Abbreviations, such as Rep., Reps., Sen., and Sens., are acceptable before one or more names in regular text.

Sen. Daniel J. Smith (R-NE) sponsored the higher education bill.

The Nebraska senator said he believed the legislation was necessary to achieve the nation's long-term goals.

Loath, loathe. An adjective, loath means "unwilling or reluctant." A verb, loathe means "to detest greatly."

He was loath to admit his misjudgment of the employee.

She loathed her job.

Long-term, short-term. Hyphenate as an adjective.

The health-care team agreed on long-term (short-term) goals involving staff in shared governance.

Loose, lose. An adjective, loose means "free" or "unattached." A verb, lose means "to part with unintentionally."

The dressing was loose again.

Do not lose the opportunity to submit your abstract.

M

Majority, plurality. Use majority to mean "more than half of an amount." Plurality means "greater" or "more than the next highest number."

When majority or plurality stands alone, use a singular verb. If a plural word follows majority of or plurality of, use either a singular or plural verb, depending on the meaning of the sentence.

> *The majority elects.*
>
> *The majority of nurses disagree with the decision.*
>
> *She won by a narrow plurality.*
>
> *His plurality was 10,000 votes.*

Male nurse. When necessary to identify a nurse by gender, the appropriate usage is male nurse, not man nurse. Avoid using man as an adjective.

Master of arts, master of science. Lowercase. Abbreviations such as MA, MS, MPH, EdM, and MBA are acceptable in professional writing. No periods are necessary, but be consistent in usage. Always use an apostrophe for "master's degree" and "master's degree program."

> *He expects to earn his master's degree in 2008.*
>
> *She graduated from the master's degree program in psychology.*

Media. Avoid the use of media to mean "a type of mass communication." Terms such as *the press, journalism, newspapers,* and *electronic press* are preferable. Media is the plural of medium.

Medical-surgical. Hyphenate rather than use a slash as in medical/surgical nursing, except when a proper name indicates otherwise.

Memorandum. The preferred plural is memorandums, but memoranda is acceptable.

Metaphor. See Figurative language.

Methodology, method. Use method to mean the plans or procedures to accomplish a goal and methodology to mean "principles referring to theoretical analysis."

He found a satisfactory method to organize his work.

The committee rejected her research because of faulty methodology.

Minority. Minority can be defined as an ethnic, religious, political, national, or other group regarded as different from the larger group of which it is a part. When referring to an ethnic, religious, political, national, or other group, substitute people of color rather than use the term minority. It is used as both a noun and an adjective.

Ruth was the first person of color to serve as president.

Modifiers. Words, phrases, or clauses in a sentence that limit or explain something are considered modifiers. Proper placement is important to avoid confusing your reader.

a. *Dangling modifiers.*

Poor: *Weighing the options carefully, a decision was made.*

Improved: *Weighing the options carefully, they decided . . .*

b. *Misplaced modifiers.*

Poor: *The patient gave the nurse an incomplete history because of her anxiety.* (Was it the patient or the nurse's anxiety?)

Improved: *Because of her anxiety, the patient gave the nurse an incomplete history.*

Money, monies. Use money, a collective noun, and avoid the plural monies.

Months. Always capitalize. Do not separate a month and year with a comma when there is no specific date. Do not abbreviate in professional writing.

He was born in January 1972.

He was born on January 28, 1972.

When listing months in tabular form, use three-letter forms without a period: *Jan, Feb, Mar, Apr, May, Jun, Jul, Aug, Sep, Oct, Nov, Dec*

More important, more importantly. Whenever possible, rephrase a sentence to avoid the use of more importantly (adverb) or more important (adjective).

> Poor: *Her report was more important than mine; more importantly, she received greater visibility.*
>
> Improved: *Her report was more timely than mine. Furthermore, she received greater visibility.*

Mr., Mrs., Ms., Messrs. Most publications omit these titles after giving the full name. Although we suggest using only the surname, follow the preferred style of the target journal. For situations in which the person has an earned doctoral degree, the use of Dr. is optional.

> *Hope Smith, PhD, and Rachel Bernini, MSN, were assigned to the case. Both Smith and Bernini agreed that it was a challenging task.*

Myriad. Myriad is a troublesome word. Most grammarians recognize its use only as an adjective meaning "a great number," such as *myriad ideas*. Modern usage, however, recognizes its use as a noun, as in *a myriad of ideas*.

N

Nationalities and races. Capitalize the proper names of nationalities, people, races, and tribes, such as *African American, American, Arab, Asian, Cherokee, Chinese, Hispanic, Jewish,* and *Native American.* Use White instead of Caucasian. See Minority.

Nauseous, nauseated. Nauseous is an adjective meaning "causing nausea." Nauseated is a verb meaning "to suffer from nausea."

> *She complained about the nauseous taste of the new medication.*
>
> *The new medicine nauseated her.*

Necessitate, require. Use necessitate, a transitive verb, to imply unavoidability. Use require, also a transitive verb, to mean "to need or to have need for."

The emergency operation necessitated a change in the staff's schedule.

His injuries required immediate surgery.

Neither, nor. Neither is almost always followed by nor. When singular, the subjects connected by neither . . . nor take a singular verb.

Neither John nor Melissa is prepared for the licensing examination.

Neither a borrower nor a lender be.

When plural, the subjects take a plural verb.

Neither the state senators nor representatives are willing to take a stand on the complicated political issue.

Neologism. A "new word." Derived from the Greek *neo* "new" and *logos* "word." All words were once neologisms so it is possible that a word first considered unacceptable might be accepted and integrated into standard language. Other neologisms flourish temporarily and eventually fade and die.

Many words began as "buzz" words, most prominently in the computer industry, and have become part of everyday speech. For example, *weblog* began in the late 1990s as a neologism, but has been shortened to form *blog,* which is accepted as a noun and a verb.

Some words emanating from other languages have been popularized, such as "bagel" (from the Yiddish word *beygel*) or *jihad* for "holy war," while others come from acronyms and abbreviations. To illustrate, *AIDS* is "acquired immune deficiency syndrome," and *laser* is an abbreviation of "light amplification by stimulated emission of radiation."

None. Means "no one, not one, or not any." Singular or plural, depending on the meaning.

Of all the concerns, none is more pressing than the credentialing quagmire. (singular)

None of the charges against her is serious. (singular)

Almost none of the professors were interviewed by the dean. (plural)

None but Debbie's greatest admirers support her election. (plural)

Not only, but also. Avoid misplacement of this pair.

Poor: *It would not only be inappropriate, but also untimely.*

Improved: *It would be not only inappropriate, but also untimely.*

The word <u>also</u> may be omitted if it does not impair the balance of the sentence.

It would be not only inappropriate, but untimely.

Nowhere, nowheres. <u>Nowheres</u> is often misused for <u>nowhere.</u> Avoid in formal writing.

Numerals. Cardinal numbers are numbers used in simple counting. Ordinal numbers indicate place, such as *second, sixth, fourth,* and so on.

Spell out cardinal numbers and ordinal numbers from one to nine; use numerals for numbers ten and above.

Abe walked six miles to the schoolhouse.

By the time he began his practice, Charlton had undergone more than 12 years of preparation.

Anna was in the fifth grade when she decided to become a teacher.

Because you must spell them out, avoid using numerals at the beginning of a sentence.

Poor: *Fifteen hundred nurse practitioners attended the workshop on women's health.*

Improved: *The workshop on women's health drew 1,500 nurse practitioners.*

In money amounts of more than 1 million, use the currency sign and spell out million, billion, and so on: $2 million, $28.5 billion. Use round numbers when appropriate.

Common fractions should be spelled out, as in *half the members, a three-fourth majority.* Use numerals for mixed fractions as in *2 1/2 hours.*

Avoid adding <u>nd</u>, <u>th</u>, <u>st</u> to dates.

> Poor: *June 2nd, March 5th, May 1st, 2004*
>
> Improved: *June 2, March 5, May 1, 2004*

Unless otherwise recommended, use Arabic numbers (1, 2, 5, 12, and so on) when citing references. Arabic numbers generally take less space and are easier to understand than Roman numbers. Suggest *Vol. 9,* not *Vol. IX.*

Nurse executive. Term generally applied to nurses in the top management position and to some holding middle management positions.

Nurse manager. A nurse heading a patient care unit who is responsible and accountable for the 24-hour management of that unit.

Nurse practitioner. Term applied to a registered nurse prepared at the master's degree level or higher who provides primary health care.

Nursing. Generally lowercase.

> *Flo decided on a career in nursing.*

O

Of. Avoid using <u>of</u> with adjectives or adverbs, such as <u>how</u> and <u>too.</u>

> Poor: *How long of a recovery do you anticipate?*
>
> *It's too complicated of a task to complete in one day.*
>
> Improved: *How long a recovery do you anticipate?*
>
> *It is too complicated a task to complete in one day.*

Office. Capitalize only when used as part of an agency's or institution's formal name. Lowercase all other uses.

> *The Oval Office of the President*
>
> *The instructor's office*

OK, Ok'd, okay, ok'ing. Use only for informal speech and writing.

On one hand, on the other hand. Use these two transitional phrases as a pair. For less wordiness, substitute <u>yet</u>, <u>but</u>, or <u>however</u>.

> Poor: *On one hand, she hoped for a favorable report. On the other hand, she knew her prognosis was guarded.*
>
> Improved: *She hoped for a favorable report but knew her prognosis was guarded.*

One. Avoid using the pronoun one as the subject of a sentence.

> Poor: *When debating an issue, one should be sure of the facts.*
>
> Improved: *Be sure of the facts when debating an issue.*

One another. Use interchangeably with <u>each other</u>.

Only. Place only <u>before</u> the word it modifies.

> *Only Mary cared about passing the test.* (Mary cared, the others did not.)
>
> *Mary cared only about passing the test.* (Mary did not care about anything but passing the test.)

Operationalize. Use sparingly. May be considered corporate or bureaucratic jargon. See <u>Verb usage: keep your verbs as verbs</u>.

Oral, verbal. Not interchangeable. <u>Oral</u> refers to the spoken word. <u>Verbal</u> refers to the spoken or written word.

> *The psychologist gave an oral promise.*
>
> *His verbal skills will take him far in life.*

Orient, orientate. Synonymous verbs meaning "to make familiar" or "to locate." Avoid <u>orientate</u>, a pretentious term, except to mean "to face or turn to the east."

Over. Use to indicate motion or a "position higher than or above another." Not interchangeable with more than.

Poor: *Cynthia Wu worked at her post for over 20 years.*

Improved: *Cynthia Wu worked at her post for more than 20 years.*

Owning to, due to. Owing to means "because of, on account of." Due to means "the result of." Owing to may be used at the beginning of a sentence meaning "because of." Due to should not be used in this way.

Owing to inclement weather, the performance was canceled.

The success of the play was due to good weather.

P

Pagination. When preparing a manuscript, begin Arabic numbering on page 2 in the upper right corner, flush with the upper margin. Do not number page 1 unless the publication requests it.

Parallelism. Refers to sentences or phrases in which the elements have the same format or relationships expressed in the same grammatical format.

He relaxes by communing on a mountaintop, snorkeling in the Bahamas, and singing in the shower.

Avoid faulty parallelism. Do not use the same grammatical form when the words or groups of words are not logical or parallel.

Poor: *The patient was asked to call the physician's secretary and an appointment would be given.*

Improved: *The patient was asked to call the physician's secretary to make an appointment.*

Parentheses and brackets. Use parentheses normally to surround numbers or letters listing items in a series: *(1) the symptoms, (2) the diagnosis.*

In the first reference to members of the U.S. Congress, always indicate the political and geographic designation, in parentheses, immediately after the name.

Sen. John Fairweather (D-CT) attended the reception.

Parentheses are also used to enclose loosely related explanations.

Brackets have little use in professional writing. Editorial remarks inserted as explanations within a quote, or a bridging phrase substituted for an omitted portion of a quote, should appear in brackets. They are used primarily for stage directions and for enclosing *[sic]* to indicate misspellings in quotes.

Her memo concluded with "Yours truley [sic], Sally Chase."

Colette [pacing]: How long must we wait?

Participles. See Verbals.

Payer, payor. Payer as "a payer of bills" is the proper usage. Many medical and nursing journals, however, use payor, a variant of payer, as their style.

People, persons. People refers to a group and implies anonymity, except when emphasizing certain individuals. Persons refers to unnamed individuals within a group.

Thousands of people attended the concert.

Luther Kean, Rozella Ford, and Dee Ferguson were among the people invited to the retreat.

Of the 50 people she invited, only 20 persons attended.

Per. A preposition. Two common meanings are "to, for, for every" and "according to."

The cardiologist recommended that Fred swim no more than one hour per day.

Per instructions of the vice president, the associate directors revised their departmental budgets.

Percent. Percent can take either a singular or plural verb, depending on its meaning. Per cent, written as two words, is obsolete.

The program director said 20 percent was too low a figure. (singular verb)

> *The medical society's statistics show that 40 percent of physicians in*
> *the state support the measure.* (plural verb)

Use the word <u>percent</u>, rather than the symbol, in formal writing except in charts, graphs, or tables. Numerals should always be used with percentages.

> Poor: *The margin of error is 15%.*
>
> Improved: *The margin of error is 15 percent.*

Percentage. Use <u>percentage</u>, rather than <u>percent</u>, to indicate a portion or amount.

> *A large percentage of the membership voted to move ahead with the*
> *hospital's new total quality management program.*
>
> *A high percentage of the patients on 4C were diagnosed with HIV.*

Periods. Use a period to end a sentence or a complete or independent thought. Also use periods with:

- initials of names (there should always be a space between initials)
  M. J. Malone

- abbreviation for the United States when used as an adjective
  U.S. Army

- abbreviations or acronyms only if they spell a word that might be mis-understood or if the abbreviation or acronym has another meeting
  I.N.A.N.E. (International Association of Nurse Editors)

Do not use periods with:

- state abbreviations
  PA, NJ, AZ

- most abbreviations or acronyms
  NLN, APHA, ANA, ASPEN

When a sentence ends with an abbreviation, use only one period.

Perk, perquisite. A <u>perquisite</u> is a benefit. Use <u>perk</u> (an abbreviation of perquisite) only in informal writing.

One of the perquisites for remaining five years was a substantial Christmas bonus.

One of the medical center's perks was free parking.

Phenomenon, phenomena. Phenomenon is singular, phenomena is plural.

Dr. Morton's introduction of sulfuric ether at Massachusetts General Hospital was considered not only an innovation but an amazing phenomenon.

The study of phenomena is an important concept in qualitative research.

Plurals. Plurals are terms composed of more than one member, set, or kind. Plurals appear in several ways.

a. common nouns. Add s or es to form plurals, as in nurses, lenses, glasses. Add es to words ending in o preceded by a consonant, as in *potatoes* and *heroes,* but not *pianos* or *mottos.* Many, but not all, words ending in y form their plurals by dropping the y and adding ies, as in *ponies, societies, deities.*

b. combined words. Usually add the s to the first word as in *sisters-in-law, Attorneys General,* or *rights-of-way.* In military titles, however, the s is usually added to the second word as in *lieutenant colonels* or *major generals.*

Several editors in chief spoke at the journalism seminar.

c. proper names. As in simple plurals, merely add an s or es. Names that end in y do not change to ie; add an s as in *Kennedys.* Exceptions include the mountain chains called the *Rockies* and *Alleghenies.* If a name ends in es or z, add es: *Joneses, Gonzalezes.*

d. numerals. Add s alone and omit the apostrophe ('). Use the closed apostrophe, however, as a contraction for decades.

1960s, size 10s, 1920s, '90s, Roaring 20s, in her 30s

e. letters. With single letters, use an apostrophe; with multiple letters, no apostrophe.

P's, q's, ABCs, IOUs, CEOs, RNs, MDs

Plus. A conjunction meaning "increased by the addition of"; a noun meaning "a positive quality"; and an adjective meaning "positive." Plus is often used as an adjective implying "large," as in *plus sizes.*

> *My salary plus benefits is acceptable.* (conjunction)
>
> *The administrator's willingness to negotiate is a plus for the institution.* (noun)
>
> *Faith's ability to communicate is a plus factor.* (adjective)

Possessives. See Apostrophe.

Practical, practicable. Use practical to mean "relating to practice in action." Use practicable to mean "capable of being done."

> *Theory followed by practical experience is highly desirable.*
>
> *The model she proposed was too complex to be practicable.*

Practicum, practicums. A practicum is a school or college course, especially in a specialized field of study, designed to give students supervised practical application of previously studied theory. The plural is practicums.

Precipitate, precipitous. As a verb, precipitate means "to bring about abruptly." As an adjective, it means "moving heedlessly." Precipitous, an adjective, means "steep," like a precipice, but it can be used to mean "hasty, rash, or sudden." It is synonymous with the adjective precipitate.

> *The patient's noncompliance precipitated an acute attack.*
>
> *It was a precipitate move to dismiss the staff.*
>
> *His precipitous decision to close the unit would have serious consequences.*

Preventive, preventative. Interchangeable, but preventive is preferred.

Previous to, prior to. Use before rather than previous to or prior to.

Primary health care. Care an individual receives at the first point of contact with the health care system, which may occur in the community, the home, or a health care facility. Emphasis is on a long-term relationship among patient, family, and practitioner.

Primary nursing. Care provided in a health care facility in which the nurse is responsible as well as accountable for the overall plan of care of an assigned patient from admission, throughout hospitalization over a 24-hour period, to discharge.

Principal, principle. As a noun, principal means "a person of rank" or a "sum of money"; as an adjective, it means "first in rank or importance." Principle, used only as a noun, is "a basic truth or rule of conduct."

> *The principal concept of her proposal lacked credibility.*
>
> *The principal closed the school because of inclement weather.*
>
> *Never compromise your principles.*

Proved, proven. Use proven as an adjective, as in *proven facts.* Use proved only as past participle of the verb to prove.

> *The results of the drug trial confirmed the company's proven results.*
>
> *The patient's comments had proved the physician's culpability.*

Q

Quality. Normally considered a noun, quality is used sparingly as an adjective, as in *quality health care.* Always acceptable when used in compound words such as *quality assurance, quality control,* and *quality point.*

Quasi. An adjective, meaning "having some resemblance usually by possession of certain attributes."

> *The National League for Nursing is a quasi-professional nursing organization.*

Quotation marks. Quotation marks are used to indicate the exact work quoted. They are not used to introduce an indirect quotation set off by that. Place periods and commas within quotation marks. Place colons and semicolons outside quotation marks.

> *Danielle's most telling comment was "the person who thinks clearly, writes clearly."*

> *She defined "burnout": a phenomenon created by overextended individuals.*

Question marks and exclamation points may come before or after quotation marks, depending on the meaning.

> *Have you ever read "The Universal Declaration of Human Rights"?*

> *As the speaker left the podium, he called out, "Hail and farewell!"*

When a paragraph of quoted material is followed by another paragraph that continues the quotation, do not end the first paragraph with an end quote ("). Begin the second paragraph with an open quote and use the end quote only at the end of the quoted material. A quotation within a direct quotation must be indicated with single quotation marks (' ').

> *Willa Faukner encouraged the students to "follow the advice of literary experts to 'write simply as the secret of good prose.'"*

Quoted material exceeding three lines in a paragraph should be indented in block form without quotation marks.

Quote, quotation. Use quotation to mean "a passage that is quoted from a speech or work." Quote is acceptable in speech, but not in formal writing. As a verb, quote means "to repeat a passage from another work."

> Poor: *The following quote illustrates my point.*

> Improved: *The following quotation illustrates my point.*

R

Raised, reared. Only humans are reared; any living thing can be raised.

Rape. Term preferred to criminal attack, criminal assault, sexual assault, and other general terms.

Regarding. Synonymous for <u>about,</u> <u>concerning,</u> or <u>on.</u>

Regardless, irregardless. <u>Irregardless</u> is not a word. Use <u>regardless</u> to mean "in spite of" or "despite."

Regime, regimen. Not interchangeable. Use <u>regime</u> to mean "a system of management" and <u>regimen</u> for "a system of therapy."

> *Case management was the accepted regime at her hospital.*
>
> *The physician ordered the patient on a low-salt, low-cholesterol regimen.*

Regretful, regrettable. Not interchangeable. Use <u>regretful</u> to mean "full of regret, sorry." <u>Regrettable</u> means "deserving regret."

> *Dr. Ross was regretful about the misunderstanding with his staff.*
>
> *The entire incident was regrettable because two of his assistants misinterpreted the order.*

Relative (to). Means "pertinent to" or "relevant to." Not synonymous with "regarding."

> Poor: *Ms. Mahoney spoke relative to the graduate program.*
>
> Improved: *Ms. Mahoney's remarks were relative to the goals of the graduate program.*

Research, study. As a noun, use <u>research</u> to mean "a scholarly inquiry or investigation." As a verb, it means "to search or investigate exhaustively." Do not use <u>research</u> as an adjective except as part of a compound term, such as <u>research grant,</u> <u>research assistant.</u> As a noun, <u>study</u> means "pursuit of knowledge." Not all studies are research, but all research involves a study. Avoid use of the redundant term <u>research study.</u>

> Poor: *She conducted her research study on patients housed in the surgical intensive care unit.*
>
> Improved: *She conducted her research (or <u>study</u>) on patients housed in the surgical intensive care unit.*

S

Saint. Abbreviate as <u>St</u>. before the name of a saint and in names of cities and other places. Exceptions exist, particularly with names of hospitals. Check the source.

Semicolon. Be careful not to overuse this punctuation mark. Use it to create a more significant break in lieu of a comma, such as in compound sentences and between independent clauses not joined by a connecting word.

> *The committee determined several issues to be explored at the nursing retreat: advancing the education base; standardizing certification; implementing the agenda for health care reform; and improving the profession's visibility.*

> *Giving injections, particularly to children, was one of Mrs. Shott's least favorite tasks; nevertheless, it became a challenge.*

Serve, service. Both mean "to provide a service" but should not be used interchangeably. People are <u>served</u>; inanimate objects are <u>serviced</u>.

> *The aide served the patient his dinner.*

> *The electrician serviced the equipment in the patient's room.*

Sexist language. Whenever possible, use the plural form to avoid the generic use of masculine or feminine pronouns. If inappropriate, employ the gender representing the majority of the group or category described. Avoid use of <u>he or she</u> or <u>his or her</u> unless a publication for which you are writing requests this usage. To avoid this usage, use plurals.

> Poor: *A health professional cannot use knowledge that he doesn't have.*

> Improved: *Health professionals cannot use knowledge that they do not have.*

Shall, will. To express simple futurity, use <u>shall</u> in the first person and <u>will</u> in the second and third person.

We (I) shall go to the hemodynamics workshop.

You (he) will go to the hemodynamics workshop.

To express determination, promise, or command, use <u>will</u> in the first person and <u>shall</u> in the second and third persons.

We will.

You shall.

Should, would. Use <u>should</u> in all persons in place of the present subjunctive. Use <u>would</u> in all persons to express determination or habitual action.

Even if I (you, she) should fail the test, the instructor would be fair.

She cautioned me, but I would have my way.

He would consult with the therapist each week to ascertain his progress.

Simile. See <u>Figurative language</u>.

Since, because. Use <u>since</u> when you wish to refer to time, otherwise use <u>because</u>.

He typed the letter on his old manual typewriter because his computer printer broke down.

The staff has been delighted since the administration decided to decentralize the nursing service to the unit level.

Sometime, sometimes. Adverbs. <u>Sometime</u> means "at an indefinite time." <u>Sometimes</u> means "upon occasion."

Oliver planned to obtain his master's degree sometime in the future.

Sometimes Oliver was sorry that he did not return to school sooner.

Split infinitives. See <u>Verbals</u>.

State. Lowercase <u>state</u> when it refers to a specific jurisdiction standing alone. Capitalize when it refers to a state's government.

Hank was concerned about environmental problems in his state.

The State of Florida applied for federal assistance to cover hurricane damage.

Stationary, stationery. Use stationary to mean "fixed, motionless," stationery to mean "writing material."

Staunch, stanch. Use staunch, an adjective, to mean "steadfast and true." Use stanch, a verb, to mean "to stop a flow of liquid, such as blood."

Stratum, strata. Strata rather than stratums is preferred as the plural of stratum. Do not use stratas.

Supine, prone. Do not confuse the meaning of these two adjectives. Supine means "face up." Prone means "face down."

Syllabus, syllabi. Use syllabi as the plural of syllabus, rather than syllabuses.

T

Techno-. Avoid this prefix for the wired age, such as *technobabble, technophile, technosavvy,* unless you are writing for a computer journal.

That, which. Relative pronouns. When used in restrictive clauses (essential for the meaning of the sentence), use that. Use which with nonrestrictive clauses (nonessential for the meaning of the sentence). Set off nonrestrictive clauses with commas.

When she attended the cardiac symposium that took place in her hometown, the event was more exciting for her.

The maximum dosage, which must not exceed 150 mg bid, still creates some serious side effects.

This, those, these, that. Demonstrative pronouns. Use sparingly.

Poor: *This is the way Dr. Stych wants the technique performed.*

Improved: *This technique is Dr. Stych's preference.*

Through, thru. A variation of <u>through</u>, the word <u>thru</u> should not be used in formal writing.

Thus, thusly. Avoid <u>thusly</u> in formal writing.

Time. Use numerals in stating a time: <u>9:20 AM</u>. Avoid using <u>9 o'clock</u>, as well as redundant terms such as <u>9:20 AM this morning</u> or <u>3:30 PM yester-</u><u>day afternoon.</u>

AM and PM can be capitals, lowercase, or set in small capitals, with or without periods, but be consistent.

To, too. <u>To</u> is a preposition showing direction. The adverb <u>too</u> means "also."

> *Doris went promptly to the luncheon.*
>
> *We have delayed a decision too long to accomplish our goals.*

Toward, towards, to. Use <u>toward</u> or <u>towards</u> to mean "in the direction of." Use <u>to</u> when you mean "in a direction toward."

> *The nurse managers walked <u>toward</u> the conference room on their way <u>to</u> rounds.*

TV. Use <u>television</u> rather than the abbreviation in professional writing.

U

Under way. Two words.

> *Planning for one new faculty member is under way.*

Unique. This word means "the only one of its kind." Not synonymous with <u>unusual.</u>

> *The practitioner–teacher role, with its components of education and practice, is a unique concept in American nursing.*

United States. Abbreviate only as an adjective in names of government agencies, such as *U.S. Department of Commerce;* in designations of highways; and in quoted material. United States takes a singular verb. The possessive is United States'.

Universal precautions. Lowercase.

Up-to-date. Hyphenate when used as an adjective.

> *Always use the most up-to-date references in your writing.*
>
> *She kept her financial records up to date on the computer.*

Usage, use. Usage refers to "habitual or preferred practices." Use shows "employment or usefulness."

> *Good writers strive to master proper language usage.*
>
> *Sheila's use of a style guide increased her chances to publish.*

Utilize, use. Utilize is overused. Substitute use whenever possible.

V

Verb agreement. Be sure to read Chapter 2, "From Principles to Practice."
   A verb always agrees with its subject, not with modifiers or introductory phrases.

> *Here come Professor Block and the teaching assistant.*
>
> *Here comes Ms. Smiley, the clinical specialist.*

A verb agrees with its subject, not the expletive there.

> *There are many reasons for Chuck Swift's promotion.*

Singular subjects joined by or or nor take singular verbs.

> *The social worker could not determine whether the child or the mother was responsible.*

Neither Lucille nor her brother was hospitalized.

When a singular and plural subject are joined by or or nor, the verb agrees with the nearest word.

The clinical coordinator does not know whether the staff nurses or the aide is responsible for the error.

The indefinite pronouns each and every, as well as compound subjects modified by each and every, take singular verbs.

Each of the therapists is bringing a recommendation.

Each bedside unit has its own computer.

Every room and suite is equipped with the latest technology.

When a pronoun is the subject, the antecedent of the relative pronoun (who, which, or that) determines the number and person of the verb.

It is I who am accountable. (I am accountable.)

It is you who deserve the praise. (You deserve the praise.)

She is one of those progressive administrators who advocate participatory management. (Administrators advocate.)

No one, anyone, everyone, someone, nobody, anybody, everybody, and somebody all require singular verbs.

No one was prepared to assign responsibility because everyone was culpable.

Verb usage.

a. *choosing the exact verb.* Good writing requires choosing exact words to convey immediately and accurately a complex idea. Weak and common verbs such as look, walk, and go can often be replaced by concrete verbs that show action more vividly and exactly. Consider these examples:

Poor: *The patient walked down the hall in an unsteady way.*

Improved: *The patient tottered (or staggered) down the hall.*

Poor: *He looked at the psychologist in an angry way.*

Improved: *He scowled (glowered, glared) at the psychologist.*

Poor: *She made funny faces as the doctor described her options.*

Improved: *She grimaced as the doctor described her options.*

b. *accentuate the positive*. Active verbs give vitality to your writing. Avoid passive voice.

Poor: *It is expected that you will follow the protocol.*

Improved: *We expect you to follow the protocol.*

Poor: *The student was reassured by her instructor's confident manner.*

Improved: *The instructor's confident manner reassured the student.*

c. *weed out weak linking verbs*. Verbs such as is, have, and other forms of to be tend to generate lazy prose and produce tedious writing. Avoid this pitfall.

Poor: *The treatment will be for six weeks and should then be effective.*

Improved: *The six-week treatment should prove effective.*

Poor: *Frances can be on the dean's list if her grades are good.*

Improved: *Frances can make the dean's list if she maintains good grades.*

d. *keep your verbs as verbs*. Maintaining the integrity of your verbs is an important principle to follow in all types of writing. Avoid the practice of converting verbs into nouns with endings such as -tion, -tize, -ance, -ability, and -able.

Poor: *Hospital officials agreed <u>on the implementation</u> of the new orientation program.*

Improved: *Hospital officials agreed <u>to implement</u> the new orientation program.*

Poor: *Don gave an unconvincing <u>explanation</u> for his tardiness.*

Improved: *Don <u>explained</u> unconvincingly his tardiness.*

Some other common examples are:

Verb	Abstract Noun
advance	advancement of
determine	determination
excite	excitability
govern	governance
use	utilization

e. *<u>avoid converting nouns into verbs</u>.* No noun appears safe from being turned into a verb, usually but not always, by the use of the suffix <u>-ize</u>. Such verbs are jargon and have no place in professional writing. The suffix <u>-ize</u> may be an easy, even lazy way to turn nouns into verbs, but many verbs formed in this manner are nothing more than bureaucratic and corporate jargon, such as *operationalize, accessorize,* and *finalize.*

Note the following examples improperly used:

Effort	*to effort to do something*
Operation	*to operationalize*
Partner	*to partner*
Strategy	*to strategize*
Transition	*to transition*
Task	*to task*
Dialog	*to dialog*
Incentive	*to incentivize*
Liaison	*to liaise*
Network	*to network*
Purpose	*to re-purpose*

f. *excessive predication*. Avoid using more verbs than necessary.

> Poor: *The visitor entered the patient's room, which was filled with flowers.*
>
> Improved: *The visitor entered the patient's flower-filled room.*

g. *understanding transitive and intransitive verbs*. A transitive verb takes a direct object. Transitive verbs demonstrate action, such as *throw the ball, failed the course,* or *dropped the bedpan.*

Intransitive verbs do not take a direct object. An intransitive verb conveys its purpose without needing an object to complement its meaning.

> *John disappeared.* (You do not disappear something.)
>
> *The storm thundered for hours.* (You do not thunder something).

Verbals. A verbal is a verb used as a noun, adjective, or adverb. A verbal may be a gerund, participle, or infinitive.

a. *gerund*. A verbal created by adding -ing to a verb; used as a noun, while conveying the meaning of a verb.

> *Editing* (from to edit) *becomes easier when using a style guide.*

b. *participle*. A verbal formed by adding -ing is a present participle. Past participles end in -d, -ed, -n, -en, or -t (unless the verb changes form altogether, such as *sung*). Participles are used as adjectives.

> *Smiling, Dorothy accepted her colleague's thanks.*
>
> *Embarrassed by her faux pas, she tried to recover her composure.*

Avoid adding -ing to popular words to produce senseless verbals.

> Poor: *dialoguing with peers*
>
> Improved: *conversing (or talking) with peers*
>
> Poor: *servicing clients*
>
> Improved: *helping clients*

c. *infinitive*. A verbal with to in front of the verb.

> *To err is human.* (subject)
>
> *Ms. Huffnagle loves to work on her computer.* (direct object)
>
> *This conference is the one to attend.* (adjective)
>
> *Nelson's disposition was difficult to tolerate.* (adverb modifying difficult)

d. *split infinitive*.
A split infinitive occurs when another word is placed between the to and the verb, such as *to always sing*.

> Poor: *Flo seemed to always make the same mistake.*
>
> Improved: *Flo always seemed to make the same mistake.*

In most situations, avoid split infinitives in formal writing, except when it might be preferred to creating an awkward construction as in the following:

> Poor: *to place carefully, to alert immediately*
>
> Improved: *to carefully place, to immediately alert*

Versus. Do not abbreviate as vs in professional writing. Use the abbreviation v when referring to court cases, as in *Smith v Davenport*.

> *It was nurses versus medical residents in the doubles tournament.*

Very, rather. Avoid using these overused adverbs to strengthen an adjective.

> Poor: *very big*
>
> Improved: *massive, huge*
>
> Poor: *rather touchy*
>
> Improved: *sensitive, ticklish*

Vice. As a prefix, the use of the hyphen is optional. The trend is to omit the hyphen.

> *vice-president, vice president*

Victim. Avoid using victim to refer to a patient with a disease or disability. See "Substitute Sensitive Language" in Chapter 4.

> Poor: *AIDS victim*
>
> Improved: *person with AIDS*

Virtually/literally. Adverbs meaning "nearly or almost entirely." Both words are often misused where no additional emphasis is necessary.

> Poor: *The procedure was virtually pain free.*
>
> Improved: *The procedure was pain free.*
>
> Poor: *He was literally demanding that he be allowed to enter.*
>
> Improved: *He was demanding that he be allowed to enter.*

Viz. See Latin derivatives.

W

Web site. Two words.

Whether. Whether implies an alternative and rarely needs to be followed by or not. See also If, whether.

Who, whom, whose, which. Relative pronouns. Use who to mean "he, she, or they."

> *Judith Flowers, who joined the firm in January, was a refreshing addition to the staff.*

Use whom to mean "him, her, or them."

> *Marion Rodriquez, whom the committee recommended, began the task immediately.*

Use whose (or of whom or of which) to express the possessive.

> *The committee, whose last recommendation was rejected by the board, supported the appointment of Ms. Rodriquez.*

Use <u>which</u> to describe an impersonal object or thing.

He was impressed by the group, which identified goals for the future.

<u>*Who, whose, which, what*</u>. As interrogative pronouns, they are used to introduce a direct or indirect question.

Who wants to go on grand rounds? (direct question)

The clinical specialist wondered who had ordered the consultation. (indirect question)

X

<u>*X ray, x-ray*</u>. Hyphenate as an adjective or transitive verb, not as a noun.

The x ray should be taken as soon as possible. (noun)

The x-ray therapy was successful. (adjective)

The technician x-rayed him at home. (verb)

Y

<u>*Years*</u>. Use numerals to express years. Because it is poor form to begin a sentence with a numeral, rework rather than spell out the numeral.

Poor: *1984 was a good year.*

Nineteen eighty-four was a good year.

Improved: *I believe 1984 was a good year.*

A good year was 1984.

Combine successive years with an en dash. Use 2004–05 rather than 2005–2006.

Her annual report covered the period 1998–99.

Use a closed apostrophe to form the shorter form of a year in more informal contexts.

The class of '99 won top honors.

Years as decades. When referring to a particular decade, it is permissible to spell out the years, for example, *the sixties, the nineties.*

Z

Zero. Write out <u>zero</u> in sentences where no other numeral is used.

> *The committee discussed zero-based budgeting.*

Use a unit of measurement when zero is written as a numeral.

> *The incidence of the disease rose from 0 percent to 6 percent in three months.*

Zip code. Acronym for Z(one) I(mprovement) P(rogram). When writing a mailing address, do not insert a comma between the state abbreviation (always in capital letters) and the zip code.

> *Hanover Falls, VT 95302-1593*

4

Be Clear and Direct: How to Avoid Redundancies, Euphemisms, and Clichés

REDUCE REDUNDANCY

Brevity is the soul of wit. . .

You've heard that one before! The great Bard knew what he was talking about. One of the first approaches to economical expression is recognizing and eliminating redundant terms. Padding, or the use of unnecessary words or phrases, clutters and obscures meaning. Trim your writing and join the other "word watchers of America." Make every word you use count. Superfluous word usage—overkill—hurts your writing.

In the following list, the words in *italics* are redundant.

a *period* of one year	consensus *of opinion*
absolutely essential	continue *on*
adequate enough	costs *the sum of*
advanced planning	cull *from*
advanced warning	each *and every*
all-inclusive	early *on*
all *of*	elaborate *on*
attached *hereto*	eliminate *completely*
basic fundamentals	enclosed *herewith*
blue *in color*	*end* result

boxlike *in shape*
complete absence
completely unanimous
connected *together*
few *in number*
final outcome
foreseeable future
full and *complete*
future plans
future prospects
generally speaking
ground rules
habitual custom
handsome *looking*
important essential
in my *best* judgment
intradermal skin tests
  (eliminate either *intradermal*
  or *skin*)
male prostate gland
many *in number*
modern hospital *of today*

endorse *on the back*
entirely completed
exact same
extremely minimal
my *own* autobiography
new record
off *of*
past experience
past history
personal opinion
*pre*planning
reason *why*
recur *again*
research *study*
revert *back*
round *in shape*
serious crisis
small *in size*
spell out *in detail*
temporary reprieve
true facts
unexpected surprise

STEER CLEAR OF EUPHEMISMS

Euphemisms are words or phrases designed to avoid using harsh, blunt, or offensive terms. Substitute the "real thing." Here are some examples:

Euphemism	Substitute
concerned	worried
deceased, passed away	died, dead
experience discomfort	hurt
frustrate	annoy, disappoint
inappropriate	wrong, untimely, inept
negative evaluation	disapproval

noncompliant	defiant
nonperformance	failure, neglect
not comfortable with	disagree, dislike
terminate	die, end

SUBSTITUTE SENSITIVE LANGUAGE

Accentuate the positive when using language to describe disabled persons; emphasize the people rather than the disability. Try to incorporate words and phrases that convey the dignity of the individual. Some examples of preferred words and phrases follow:

developmentally disabled
disabled
hearing impaired
mentally/emotionally disabled
mentally restored
mentally impaired
multihandicapped
nondisabled
persons with AIDS
persons with cerebral palsy
persons with disabilities
persons with paraplegia
seizure
visually impaired
wheelchair-user

Poor: *Ms. Davis is a crippled woman confined to a wheelchair.*

Improved: *Ms. Davis is a woman with a disability who uses a wheelchair.*

Poor: *The victims in the rehabilitation program were afflicted with a variety of problems.*

Improved: *Participants in the rehabilitation program included individuals with disabilities due to cerebral palsy, war injuries, and alcohol abuse.*

ELIMINATE TRITENESS

Trite expressions or clichés are familiar combinations of words, often-used quotations, and worn-out figures of speech. They should be replaced. Here are some examples:

acid test
after all is said and done
age before beauty
all that glitters is not gold
all work and no play
ball park figure
(with) bated breath
better late than never
blue in the face
blue sky
blushing bride
bolt from the blue
bottom line
breathe a sigh of relief
bright and shining faces
brown as a berry
budding genius
chip off the old block
clear as a bell
cool as a cucumber
cradle of the deep
dead as a doornail
diamond in the rough
dull thud
fast and furious
few and far between
(the) finer things in life
get off your high horse
green with envy
heart of gold
humble origin
irony of fate

it stands to reason
know-how
leaps and bounds
method in your (his, my) madness
ominous silence
path to success
proud possessor
quiet as a mouse
rears its ugly head
road of life
sadder but wiser
sick as a dog
slow as molasses
sly as a fox
smart as a whip
think tank
(the) time of my life
tired but happy
touch base
wine, women, and song
with all due respect

5

Harness the Potential of Computers and the Internet

Most, if not all, writers today use computers and can capitalize on a variety of built-in tools standard in most word-processing programs, as well as add-on software programs. *Although new and sophisticated software is continually being created, do not expect computer software to substitute for a good style manual, dictionary, or English composition text.*

GRAMMAR CHECKERS

Software in this category analyzes words within the context of the sentences in which they are used. The program highlights errors and suggests corrections. Most programs have pull-down menus for rules on grammar and style. In some cases, you can customize the checker to your particular field of writing, such as technical, business, fiction, legal, and so on.

Most software programs can identify and correct problems in the following areas:

abbreviations
adverb, adjective usage
archaic usage
colloquial expressions
double negatives
end-of-sentence prepositions
jargon
long sentences

 passive voice
 pronoun cases
 punctuation and spelling errors
 redundancies
 split infinitives
 subject and verb agreement
 wordiness

Many grammar checkers and software programs such as Microsoft Word also analyze a document, review usage of passive voice, and study readability and writing level, sentence and paragraph length, and other areas.

Using a popular search engine, we turned up myriad Web sites promoting grammar and writing software programs, mostly sold to add on to Microsoft Word. Remember these Web sites are marketing tools, so be wary when researching products. One program sold itself as "a software tool . . . that applies powerful editing techniques to improve clarity and readability in a fraction of the time it takes to edit without assistance." Another program billed itself as "the best word processing add-on on the market. It teaches you to write in the style of top authors and journalists." "The best writer's software suite on the market today. . . . [I]t is the most complete book-writing software suite today," touted another.

If you decide to purchase software for grammar, style, or spell checking, heed the motto "buyer beware." Take advantage of free trial downloads if possible, or check out local computer software supercenters to see if they provide a lab for testing. Although software programs can assist writers, their impact is negligible compared to the resources available on the Internet.

THE INTERNET REVOLUTION

Born in the 1960s as a network connecting government computers to a small group of universities doing Defense Department business, the Internet expanded to the general public in the 1990s when the National Science Foundation ended its sponsorship of the Internet system. All traffic switched to commercial networks such as AOL, Prodigy, and CompuServe; but when Microsoft launched Windows 98 with an integrated browser, Internet usage exploded.

As the computer industry has grown and expanded, the Internet has evolved. Video and audio streaming and telephone service are commonplace. On the horizon looms Internet television.

How will the Internet continue to expand and change? That remains to be seen; but it is safe to say the Internet remains the frontier for aspiring writers to obtain style and grammar resources.

THE RESOURCES OF THE WORLD WIDE WEB

Surfing Web Sites

As an aspiring author, you can use the Internet to access different nursing and health journals and select the most appropriate one for your article. You can usually view the latest issue, possibly abstracts of articles, a table of contents, background on the journal, and so on. Some journal Web sites provide guidelines for authors or direct you on how to obtain a copy. You can also surf journal Web sites to determine if your idea is unique.

Using Search Engines

Search engines, Web sites that let users locate information on the World Wide Web, can help you research your article. Search engines work by entering keywords to find Web sites or locate documents that contain the information the user is seeking.

At the time of publication, Google (*www.google.com*) is perhaps the most well known search engine, spawning a neologism, the verb "to google," meaning to look up on the Web. Other search engines include Yahoo (*www.yahoo.com*), the oldest Web directory, launched in 1994; Lycos (*www.lycos.com*); Ask.com (*www.ask.com*); AOL Search (*http://aolsearch.aol.com*—internal or *http://search.aol.com*—external); MSN (*www.msn.com*); and Clusty (*http://clusty.com*), which clusters its searches by topic, sources, or URL. Check out the SearchEngineWatch Web site for complete lists and ratings (*http://searchenginewatch.com*).

Knowing the Source

Proceed cautiously when using online resources. Be sure you can trust the source before you use its information. A "blog" is a Web log or an online personal journal or series of postings on any subject whose authors are called "bloggers." Be wary of bloggers who claim to be experts in any field, but especially style and grammar.

One search engine produced more than 1.6 million "hits" for the words *guide, grammar,* and *style.* With such vast reach, dangers—from questionable information sources to computer viruses—abound. For example, one online grammar service that said it would help the reader get A's on a term paper had several misspelled words on its own Web site!!

University Web sites, on the other hand, can be excellent, reliable resources. One example, Brown University Graduate School's Writing Center, links to reputable indices, grammar Web sites, books, and Web sites providing help in citing sources and documentation and preparing annotations and annotated bibliographies (*www.brown.edu/Student_Services/Writing_Center/style.htm*).

Many important reference books have online versions. Bartleby.com (*www.bartleby.com*) provides access to reference books online, such as the *American Heritage Dictionary, Roget's International Thesaurus, Bartlett's Familiar Quotations, Gray's Anatomy, Bulfinch's Mythology, The King James Version of the Bible,* and many more. (See Appendix E.)

Writers can use the Internet to augment their own library of resources, such as this *Health Professionals Style Manual.* You also need a recent edition of a good dictionary, such as the *American Heritage Dictionary* or *Merriam-Webster's Collegiate Dictionary* or *Merriam-Webster Unabridged Dictionary,* and *Roget's Thesaurus.* Other important resources are listed in References for Further Reading at the back of this book.

AVOIDING PLAGIARISM

Merriam-Webster's Collegiate Dictionary defines *to plagiarize* as "to steal and pass off the ideas or words of another as one's own" or to "use another's production without crediting the source."

Whether caused by sloppy note taking and documentation or outright "pirating," plagiarism is wrong; you must preserve your own integrity as well as respect of the works of others. Unfortunately, the Internet has made plagiarism easier than ever before. An author can copy a sentence, paragraph, an entire article, and even graphics with just a few clicks of the mouse. Yet the same principles followed in printed communication must apply to the Internet. Plagiarism is always inexcusable.

Recognizing the delicate balance between the rights of copyright holders and the public, the American Library Association outlined the public's right to access information in electronic formats. According to the ALA statement (1995), without infringing copyright, the public has a right to expect:

- to read, listen to, or view publicly marketed copyrighted material privately, on site or remotely;
- to browse through publicly marketed copyrighted material;
- to experiment with variations of copyrighted material for fair use purposes, while preserving the integrity of the original;
- to make or have made for them a first-generation copy for personal use of an article or other small part of a publicly marketed copyrighted work or a work in a library's collection for such purpose as study, scholarship, or research; and
- to make transitory copies if ephemeral or incidental to a lawful use and if retained only temporarily.

The concern about online plagiarism and theft of content spawned a Web site, called Copyscape, that "finds sites that have copied your content without permission, as well as those that have quoted you." The site provides help for avoiding plagiarism, such as printing banners on Web sites and including copyright notices on each page of a Web site (*www.copyscape.com*).

The United States Copyright Office has information covering the registration of original works online such as Web sites. (See *Circular 66, Copyright Registration for Online Works* from the United States Copyright Office.) Copyright registration of a Web site, however, must be reregistered every time the site is significantly updated.

Avoid plagiarism by:

- using quotations to cite any material that is taken verbatim. Be especially careful when taking notes to ensure you do not mistake a direct quote for your writing.
- documenting your sources meticulously.
- paraphrasing material while being cautious not to just change a few words. Indiana University at Bloomington's Writing Tutorial Service advises students to "read over what you want to paraphrase

carefully; cover up the text with your hand, or close the text so you can't see any of it . . . Write out the idea in your own words without peeking."

- comparing your paraphrased material to the original to make sure you have not accidentally used the source's words.

UNDERSTANDING E-MAIL ETIQUETTE

Cheaper than a phone call and faster than overnight mail, electronic mail or e-mail is rapidly becoming the preferred method of written communication. E-mail offers an ease and immediacy unimagined only a few years ago. What you save on costs, however, can cost you in other ways. Just because the turnaround time can be almost immediate, do not treat e-mail communication lightly.

Many e-mail "how to" books assert conversational writing is acceptable in composing an e-mail. We disagree. Because you are judged by how you express yourself, professional or business communication should never be careless or poorly constructed. The rules of grammar, spelling, style, and usage contained in this book apply whether you are writing an article for publication or an e-mail.

E-mail, however, does have some particularities. Because of its spontaneity, for example, many people are uninhibited in expressing their feelings, often in a less-than-tactful manner. "Flaming," an inflammatory remark or message, is the result of firing back a message too quickly without waiting to calm down before responding.

The speed of e-mail has also spawned practices to save time. Lazy writers set the Caps Lock and type in ALL CAPS or use all lowercase letters rather than using the Shift key. Typing in ALL CAPS is called "shouting" in e-mail parlance. Reading ALL CAPS or all lowercase is not only annoying for the recipient, it makes your message difficult to read and understand.

To save a few keystrokes, many e-mail writers also use a list of abbreviations such as BBL for "be back later," LOL for "laughing out loud," or IMO for "in my opinion." Also beware of the temptation to punctuate your e-mail with "smileys," or visual shorthand of facial expressions such as ☺ or :—) for Happy, or ☹ or :—(for Sad. "Smileys" and abbreviations are no more than e-mail slang and have no place in business communication.

CONCLUSION

This review of editorial and Internet resources demonstrates the array of assistance available to writers. Software programs can catch spelling and writing errors for you, but do not be shortsighted. Although helpful, most programs have imperfections. With a grammar checker, for example, a computer often flags errors where none exists, failing, in many cases, to find the correct subject and verb of a sentence. Furthermore, such programs tend to call every complex sentence a "run-on" sentence.

An article in *USA Today* on July 15, 2002 quotes Dene Grigar, an assistant professor of English at Texas Women's University in Dallas. She believes grammar checkers "help to clear up errors that students don't mean to make," but she warned that "grammar checkers can also intimidate some students who have not developed a personal style (or voice) or do not have confidence in their writing." The author worries that grammar checkers repress a student's creativity and serve as a crutch for those without good grammar, while acknowledging there are those who find them useful.

Spell checkers too have their limitations. Often a program highlights a word, indicates that it is not in the dictionary, and suggests alternatives. What this might mean, however, is that the word in question does not exist in that particular software program's dictionary. Some spell checkers may overlook errors such as using "to" when "too" is correct. Not all spell checkers test grammar; as long as the word is spelled correctly, the program is happy.

As a health professional eager to improve your writing, wisely use existing software and Internet resources. Be mindful that these options offer no promise of enhancing your creativity or assisting in the development of your own style. View these aids primarily as adjuncts to the writing skills you must acquire through practice and the use of sound resources on composition and style. These are the best ways to be your own editor.

Appendix A

Common Abbreviations and Acronyms in Health Care

Although people tend to confuse abbreviations and acronyms, the terms are not synonymous. An abbreviation is a shortened form of a written word or phrase. Examples include *APHA (American Public Health Association)* and *CPR (cardiopulmonary resuscitation)*. An acronym is a word formed from the initial or key letter or letters of each of a series of words. *RUGS (research utilization groups)* and *MAP (mean arterial pressure)* are classified as acronyms. Acronyms may consist of adjoining letters to make them more pronounceable.

The listing below combines abbreviations and acronyms, including the more common terms used by health professionals.

ABBREVIATIONS AND ACRONYMS IN THE NURSING AND HEALTH FIELD

ABE	acute bacterial endocarditis
ABS	acute brain syndrome
ACLS	advanced cardiac life support
ACT	added compensatory time
ACVD	acute cardiovascular disease
A & D	admission and discharge
AD	admitting diagnosis
ADC	average daily census
ADHC	adult day health care
ADL	activities of daily living
AD LIB	freely

ADN	associate degree in nursing
ADP	automatic data processing
ADR	actual death rate
ADR	adverse drug reaction
ADS	alternative delivery system
ADT	admission/discharge/transfer
AEC	at earliest convenience
AIDS	acquired immune deficiency syndrome
AL	arterial line
ALC	allowable limit of care
ALC	alternate levels of care
ALOH	average length of hospitalization
ALOS	average length of stay
ALS	advanced life support
AMA	against medical advice
AMI	acute myocardial infarction
AND	administratively necessary days
ANDA	abbreviated new drug application
ANOV	analysis of variance
AOB	adjusted occupied bed
A & P	assessment and plans
APG	ambulatory patient groups
A/R	apical/radial
ASAP	as soon as possible
ASF	ambulatory surgical facility
ATLS	advanced trauma life support
AWD	absent without discharge
BB	blood bank
BC	board certified
BID	twice daily
BLS	basic life support
BM	bone marrow
BM	bowel movement
BMR	basal metabolic rate
BMT	bone marrow transplant
BP	bed pan
BP	blood pressure

BR	bed rest
BRN	baccalaureate program for registered nurse
BRN	board of registered nursing (state specific)
BRP	bathroom privileges
BSN	bachelor of science in nursing
BSN	bowel sounds normal
BT	bedtime
BU	burn unit
C	certified
CA	carcinoma (or cancer)
CABG	coronary artery bypass graft
CAI	computer assisted instruction
CAPD	continuous ambulatory peritoneal dialysis
CAR	computer assisted retrieval
CAT	computerized adaptive testing
CBC	complete blood count
CBF	cerebral blood flow
CBVI	computer-based video instruction
CC	chief complaint
CC	conventional care
CC	critical care
CCP	comprehensive care plan
CCU	coronary care unit
CCU	critical care unit
CD	cardiovascular disease
CDU	chemical dependency unit
CE	continuing education
CEA	cost-effective analysis
CEO	chief executive officer
CEU	continuing education unit
CFO	chief financial officer
CHC	community health center
CHCP	coordinated home care program
CHI	consumer health information

CHIP	comprehensive health insurance plan
CHN	community health network
CIO	chief information officer
CIS	computer information service
CM	case management
CM	case mix
CMI	case mix index
CMP	comprehensive medical plan
CNAA	certified nursing administrator advanced
CNE	chief nurse executive
CNM	certified nurse-midwife
CNP	community nurse practitioner
CNS	clinical nurse specialist
C/O	complaint of
COO	chief operating officer
COI	cost of illness
CON	certificate of need
COPD	chronic obstructive pulmonary disease
CPM	continuous passive motion
CPO	continuous pulse oximetry
CPR	cardiopulmonary resuscitation
CPU	central processing unit
CQI	continuous quality improvement
CRF	case report form
CRNA	certified registered nurse anesthetist
CRT	cardiac resuscitation team
CSPS	corporate strategic planning system
CSR	central supply room
CSW	clinical social worker
CT	computerized axial tomography
CVL	central venous line
CVP	central venous pressure
D/A	date of admission
D/C	discontinue

DD	dual degree
DDS	doctor of dental surgery
DHS	duration of hospital stay
DNA	deoxyribonucleic acid
DNA	district nurses association
DNI	do not intubate
DNR	do not resuscitate
DNS	doctor of nursing science
DNSc	doctor of nursing science
DOA	date of admission
DOA	dead on arrival
DON	director of nursing
DOQ	desired order quantity
DP	data processing
DR	delivery room
DRG	diagnosis related group
DRS	data retrieval system
DSN	doctor of science in nursing
E & A	evaluate and advise
ECF	extended care facility
ECG	electrocardiography
ECT	electroconvulsive therapy
ECU	extended care unit
ED	emergency department
EdD	doctor of education
EDP	electronic data processing
EDR	expected death rate
EEG	electroencephalography
EEO	equal employment opportunity
EKG	electrocardiography
EMT	emergency medical team
EOC	episode of care
ER	emergency room
ESRD	end stage renal disease
FAAN	fellow of the American Academy of Nursing
FFS	fee for service
FHC	family health center

FHIP	family health insurance plan
FI	fiscal intermediary
FNP	family nurse practitioner
FTE	full-time equivalent
FUO	fever of unknown origin
FY	fiscal year
GN	graduate nurse
GNP	gerontologic (geriatric) nurse practitioner
GR	grand rounds
GRE	graduate record examination
HB	hospital-based
HBO	health benefits organization
HBP	hospital-based physician
HBV	hepatitis B virus
HC	health care
HCD	health care delivery
HH	home hyperalimentation
HHA	home health agency
HHA	home health aide
HHC	home health care
HIP	health insurance plan
HIS	home information system
HIV	human immunodeficiency virus
HMO	health maintenance organization
HN	head nurse
HO	house officer
HOPA	hospital-based organ procurement agency
HP	health professional
HP	house physician
HPN	home parenteral nutrition
HPPD	hours per patient day
HPR	hospital peer review
HR	hospital record
HSC	health science center
HSI	health status index
IC	intensive care

ICF	intermediate care facility
ICP	intercranial pressure
ICU	intensive care unit
IDS	interactive data system
I/O	intake/output
IV	intravenous
IVP	intravenous pyleogram
KCF	key clinical finding
MAP	mean arterial pressure
MASH	mobile army surgical hospital
MBA	master of business administration
MC	managed care
MCH	maternal and child health
MCN	maternal child nursing
MD	doctor of medicine
MDC	major diagnostic category
MDS	minimum data set
MHA	master of health administration
MI	myocardial infarction
MIC	maternal and infant care
MICU	medical intensive care unit
MIS	management information system
MIS	medical information system
MPH	master of public health
MPP	Medicare-participating physician
MPS	multiphasic screening
MR	management reviews
MR	mental retardation
MRA	multiple regression analysis
MRI	magnetic resonance imaging
MSDS	material safety data sheet
MSN	master of science in nursing
MSW	master of social work
NA	not admitted
NA	notice of admission
NA	nursing assistant (or aide)
NCLEX	National Council Licensure Examination

NFP	not for profit
NG	nasogastric
NICU	neonatal intensive care unit
NICU	neurosurgical intensive care unit
NIS	nursing information system
NM	nurse manager
NMIS	nursing management information system
NNP	neonatal nurse practitioner
NP	nurse practitioner
NPO	nothing by mouth
NRC	nursing resource cluster
NSA	nursing service administrator
NSAIDS	nonsteroidal anti-inflammation drugs
NTA	nurse training act
NTBR	not to be resuscitated
OBS	organic brain syndrome
OCU	outpatient care unit
OD	organizational development
OJT	on-the-job training
OOB	out of bed
OPA	organ procurement agency
OPD	outpatient department
OPS	outpatient surgery
OR	operating room
OR	organ recovery
OTC	over the counter
OTR	registered occupational therapist
PA	physician's assistant
PAC	political action committee
PAP	patient assessment program
PAR	postanesthesia room
PARU	postanesthesia recovery unit
PCC	patient care clinician
PD	patient day
PDR	*Physician's Desk Reference*
PEC	patient education coordinator

PET	positron emission tomography
PGP	prepaid group practice
PHC	primary health care
PhD	doctor of philosophy
PHO	physician hospital organization
PNP	pediatric nurse practitioner
PNS	psychiatric nursing specialist
PPO	preferred provider organization
PPS	prospective payment system
PR	peer review
PRO	peer review organization
PRS	prospective reimbursement system
PSDA	patient self-determination act
PT	physical therapist
PTA	prior to admission
PTCA	percutaneous transluminal coronary angioplasty
QA & I	quality assurance and improvement
QAP	quality assurance program
QC	quality circle
QD	every day
QHS	every hour of sleep
QPC	quality of patient care
QPM	every night
QUID	four times a day
QWL	quality of work life
RC	referred care
R & D	research and development
RD	registered dietitian
RFI	request for information
RFP	request for proposal
RIMS	relative intensity measures
RM	risk management
RN	registered nurse
RNC	registered nurse certified
RNLP	registered nurse, license pending
R & R	rest and recuperation/relaxation
RR	recovery room

RT	respiratory therapist
RUGS	research utilization groups
RVS	relative value scales
RVU	relative value unit
SBE	subacute bacterial endocarditis
SBN	state board of nursing
SCU	special care unit
SG	Surgeon General
SI	seriously ill
SICU	surgical intensive care unit
SN	staff nurse
SNA	state nurses association
SNF	skilled nursing facility
SO	significant other
SOC	standard of care
SOI	severity of illness
SOP	standard operating procedure
SP	standard performance
SPA	state planning agency
SVCS	superior vena cava syndrome
SW	social worker
TC	transplant center
TID	three times daily
TLC	tender loving care
TPN	total parenteral nutrition
TQM	total quality management
TR	turnover rate
TRO	temporary restraining order
TT	turnover time
U & A	up and about
UCRS	utilization control reporting system
UCS	usual and customary service
UD	unit dose
UOS	units of service
UR	utilization review
URI	upper respiratory infection
VNA	visiting nurse association
VNS	visiting nurse service

VP	vice president
VS	vital signs
WCH	women and children's health
WL	workload
WNL	within normal limits
YACP	young adult chronic patient
YTD	year-to-date
ZBB	zero-based budgeting
ZPG	zero population growth

SELECTED ABBREVIATIONS OF NURSING ORGANIZATIONS

AAAN	American Academy of Ambulatory Nurses
AACN	American Association of Colleges of Nursing
AACN	American Association of Critical Care Nurses
AAHN	American Association for the History of Nursing
AAMCN	American Association of Managed Care Nurses
AAN	American Academy of Nursing
AANA	American Association of Nurse Anesthetists
AANA	American Association of Nurse Attorneys
AAOHN	American Association of Occupational Health Nurses
ABNS	American Board of Nursing Specialties
ACNM	American College of Nurse-Midwives
ACNP	American College of Nurse Practitioners
AFNC	Air Force Nurse Corps

AHNA	American Holistic Nurses Association
ANA	American Nurses Association
ANC	Army Nurse Corps
ANF	American Nurses Foundation
ANIA	American Nursing Informatics Association
ANNA	American Nephrology Nurses Association
AONE	American Oraganization of Nurse Executives
AORN	Association of Operating Room Nurses
APN	Alliance for Psychosocial Nursing
APNA	American Psychiatric Nursing Association
APRN	Association of Perioperative Registered Nurses
ARN	Association of Rehabilitation Nurses
AWHONN	Association of Women's Health, Obstetric and Neonatal Nurses
COGFNS	Commission on Graduates of Foreign Nursing Schools
ENA	Emergency Nurses Association
FNS	Frontier Nursing Service
GSA	Gerontological Society of America
HPNA	Hospice & Palliative Nurses Association
ICN	International Council of Nurses
INS	Intravenous Nurses Society
NCSBN	National Council of State Boards of Nursing
NINR	National Institute of Nursing Research
NLN	National League for Nursing
NNC	Navy Nurse Corps

NOADN	National Organization for Associate Degree Nursing
NSNA	National Student Nurses Association
ONS	Oncology Nursing Society
SGNA	Society of Gastroenterology Nurses and Associates
SPN	Society of Pediatric Nurses
STTI	Sigma Theta Tau International
VNAA	Visiting Nurses Associations of America

Appendix B

Commonly Misspelled Words

Writers need to be meticulous about their spelling when preparing any written work. Do not be hampered by spelling errors, which can be a source of irritation particularly to editors and teachers. Careless language can indicate careless thinking. When in doubt, always consult a dictionary.

Here is a list of words commonly misspelled in professional writing:

accidentally
accommodate
acknowledgment
acute care (noun)
acute-care (adjective)
aegis
aftercare
afterward (not afterwards)
all right (not alright)
ambiance
amid (not amidst)
among (not amongst)
anonymity
bed linen (two words)
beginning
benefited, benefiting
bona fide
byproduct
canceled
cannot
caregiver

caseload
case mix
case mix index
child rearing (noun)
child-rearing (adjective)
commitment
committable
committed
computer-assisted instruction
consensus
corollary
corroborate
cost-effective (adjective)
course work
credentialing
criterion, criteria
cross section (noun)
cross-section (adjective)
data bank
database
day care
decision making (noun)
decision-making (adjective)
degree-granting
dichotomy
downtime
eighth
embarrassed
enforce
entry level (noun)
entry-level (adjective)
existence
extended care facility
field work
fieldwork (military usage only)
flow chart (preferred) (noun)
flow-chart (verb)
foci (plural)

focused
forehead
foreword
fulfillment
fundraising (preferred)
grass roots
hands-on
handwashing
holistic
home health aide
home health care
immediately
impatient
in-depth (adjective)
in-house (adjective)
joint faculty
judgment
Kardex (proper noun)
knowledge
leisure
liaison
licensure
lifeless
life-sized
lifestyle (noun)
life support (noun)
life-support (adjective)
line item (noun)
line-item (adjective)
line-support (adjective)
long-standing
lower-division
low-key
melee
naïve
naïveté
ninety
nonfat

nonmember

nonnurse

nonprofit

occurred

ongoing

online (noun)

on-line (adjective)

on-site

outnumber

paradigm

parallel

policymaker

policymaking

printout

privilege

programmed

programming

prophecy (noun)

prophecies (plural)

prophesy (verb)

prostate

questioned

questioning

questionnaire

quid-pro-quo

range-of-motion

rank and file (noun)

rank-and-file (adjective)

recurrence

respondent

rhythm

role playing (noun)

second-guess

seize

self-care

shining

shortfall

short-run (adjective)

side effect
skeptic
spreadsheet
step-down (adjective)
synonymous
tenure-track (adjective)
third party
thus (not thusly)
time-and-motion
toward (not towards)
tragedy
traveled
traveling
under way (adverb)
underway (adjective)
upper-division
well-being (noun)
well-baby clinic
word processing (noun)
word-processing (adjective)
work force
workload
workout
workplace
workup
write-off
write-up

Appendix C

Using Prefixes and Suffixes

A general rule with prefixes and suffixes is do not use hyphens unless they serve a purpose. Compound words, however, tend to cause writing and editing problems. Are they closed or hyphenated? Or separate words? Are they treated differently as a noun than as an adjective?

Here are some principles to guide you, although exceptions exist.

WHEN TO HYPHENATE

1. Using a compound word as an adjective to avoid confusing the reader:

   fast-moving train

2. Using a phrase as an adjective preceding the term it modifies:

   to-be-recalled documents

3. Ending a prefix with a vowel followed by a word beginning with the same vowel:

   anti-inflammatory, pre-eminent, pre-election

4. Following a prefix with a word that is capitalized:

   anti-American, post-Friday, post-June 9

5. Forming a compound word with the number as the first element preceding the term it modifies:

10th-grade student, third-generation physician

6. Using the prefix *co* to form a noun, adjective, or verb that refers to an occupation or status:

co-chairperson

WHEN NOT TO HYPHENATE

1. Using the prefix *non:*

nonviolent, nonpartisan, nonsignificant, nonnursing

2. Using a word formed with the suffix *wise* when it means "in the direction of" with regard to:

clockwise, dollarwise

3. Using a word formed with the suffix *like* unless the letter would be in triple:

skill-like, childlike

Our choice of appropriate prefixes and suffixes follows below. For any omissions, we suggest that you consult a dictionary.

Prefixes: Affixes Before a Word to Produce a Derivative Word

Ante

ante-Christianity
antebellum
antedate
antediluvian
anteroom

Anti

anti-American
anti-inflammatory
anti-inflation
anti-intellectual
antihypertensive
antisocial
antitoxin
antitrust

Bi

biennial
bifocal
bilateral
bilingual
bipartisan
bivalent
biweekly

By

bylaw
byline
bypass
byproduct

Co

co-author
co-chairperson
co-editor
co-host
co-op
co-sponsor
coeducation
coexist
cooperate

coordinate
coworker

Cross

cross-country
cross-examine
cross-purpose
cross-reference
crossbred
crosscut
crosstown

Dis

disabled
disaffection
disservice

Extra

extracranial
extracurricular
extramarital
extraterrestrial

Half

half-baked
half-hour
half-life
half-truth
halfhearted
halftime
halfway
half brother
half dollar
half size

Hyper

hypercritical
hyperemia
hyperphysical
hyperspace

In

in-group
in-house
in-law
inbound
infrared
infield
inpatient

Mid

mid-America
mid-Atlantic
mid-1990
mid-90s
midlife
midsemester
midterm
Midwest

Multi

multidisciplinary
multifaceted
multilateral
multimillionaire
multiphase

Non

nonaligned
noncontroversial

nonpartisan
nonviolent
nonworking

Over

overachiever
overdue
overeager
overrate
override
oversensitive

Post

post-baccalaureate
post-mortem
post-2005
postbellum
postdate
postdoctoral
postgraduate
postoperative
posttest

Pre

pre-conference
pre-election
pre-establish
pre-exist
pre-experiment
pre-Hellenic
pre-malignant
prearrange
preheat

Pro

pro-American
pro-environment
proactive
progovernment
prorated
prowar

Re

re-emphasize
re-establish
re-use
reconsider
reevaluate
rethink
reunify

Self

self-acting
self-address
self-defeating
self-employ
self-esteem
self-evident
self-paced

Semi

semi-independent
semi-invalid
semiannual
semifinal
semiofficial

Sub

subaverage
subcommittee
subcontract
subtotal

Super

superagency
supercharge
superhighway
superpower
supertanker

Trans

trans-Atlantic
trans-configuration
trans-dichloro-ethylene
transcontinental
transcutaneous
transsexual

Un

un-American
unarmed
unbelievable
unnecessary
unsolved
unsterile

Under

underdog
underestimate

underrepresented
underused

Wide

wide-angle
wide-awake
wide-eyed
wide-open
widesought
widespread

Suffixes: Affixes at the End of a Word to Produce a Derivative Word

In

break-in
cave-in
walk-in
write-in

Like

bill-like
shell-like

Off

send-off
stop-off
cutoff
playoff
standoff
takeoff

Over

carryover
changeover
makeover
rollover
turnover

Out

cop-out
fade-out
fallout
pullout
turnout
walkout

Up

close-up
follow-up
breakup
buildup
checkup
markup

Wise

health-wise
tax-wise
clockwise

Appendix D

Common Proofreader's Marks

Mark	Explanation	Example
‖	Align/No indent	‖ Cleveland is
⌇	Boldface	⌇ Cleveland
e/	Correction	Cleveland e/
⌒	Close up space	Cleve⌒land
⊆	Capital letter	cleveland
≡	Capitalize	Cleveland
⌀	Delete	Cleveland
$\frac{1}{M}$	Indent 1 em	$\frac{1}{M}$ Cleveland is the
$\frac{2}{M}$	Indent 2 ems	$\frac{2}{M}$ Cleveland is the
$\frac{3}{M}$	Indent 3 ems	$\frac{3}{M}$ Cleveland is the

Mark	Explanation	Example
$\hat{2}$	Inferior (subscript) figures (symbols)	CO_2 $co\hat{2}$
$\#$	Insert space	Clevelanḓthe $\#$
$\overset{\vee}{}$	Insert apostrophe	Clevelands riverfront
$\hat{}$	Insert a comma	Cleveland˄Ohio
$£/Ʒ/$	Insert brackets	Cleveland˄Ohio˄ $£/Ʒ/$
$\{/\}/$	Insert parentheses	Cleveland˄Ohio˄ $\{/\}/$
$\odot$	Insert a period	Cleveland, Ohio⊙
$\wedge$	Insert information	Clev˄land e˄
$\overset{\alpha}{\vee}$ $\overset{\prime\prime}{\vee}$	Insert quotation marks	˅I like Cleveland˅ $\overset{\alpha}{\vee}$ $\overset{\prime\prime}{\vee}$
stet	Let it stand	Cleveland is the (*stet*)
$\smile$	Less space	Characteristic‿of
$\underset{}{\smile}$	Lower	Cleveland ⌣is⌡
lc	Lowercase letter	Cleveland /ɪs *lc*
lc	Lowercase letters	CL/EVELAND *lc*
$\sqsubset$	Move left	⊏| Cleveland
$\sqsupset$	Move right	⊐Cleveland |
$¶$	New paragraph	the last. Cleveland is the $¶$
no $¶$	No new paragraph, run in	the last. ⊃ ⊂Cleveland is the *no* $¶$

Mark	Explanation	Example
⌐⌐	Raise	Cleveland ⌐is⌐
ital	Set in italics	Cleveland *ital*
rom	Set in roman type	Cleveland *rom*
=	Small capitals	Cleveland
⁴∨	Superior (superscript) figures (footnotes)	Cleveland is the largest ⁴∨
tr	Transpose	Cleveland the is *tr*
tr	Transpose in order	Cleveland capital the is not (1 5 4 2 3)
wf	Wrong font	Cleveland *wf*

Appendix E

Electronic Resources

www.apastyle.org The online version of the *Publication Manual of the American Psychological Association*

www.m-w.com The online version of the Merriam-Webster dictionaries.

www.bartleby.com/reference The online version of *Roget's International Thesaurus, American Heritage Dictionary, Columbia Encyclopedia, Bartlett's Familiar Quotations, The Columbia Guide to Standard American English, The King James Version of the Bible, Bulfinch's Mythology,* and more

www.brown.edu/Student_Services/Writing_Center/style.htm Online links to reputable Web sites providing assistance to writers

www.press.uchicago.edu Online information from *The Chicago Manual of Style*

www.columbia.edu/acis/bartleby/strunk/ Online version of *The Elements of Style*

Appendix F

Referencing

By documenting a written work, you credit the source. You add to the credibility of the discussion in progress because, by their very nature, citations show the effectiveness of the supporting evidence. A listing of endnotes consistent with references in the text will enable the reader to retrieve and use the sources.

If you want to publish, obtain the style requirements of the journals or publishing companies where you intend to send your work. Check the journals in the health care arena; most of them carry guidelines that appear on a regular basis and clearly identify reference specifications. In addition, Web sites of the organizations may provide guidelines. You may also write to or e-mail a publication for the information.

Although a number of editors follow the general pattern of academia, which favors the *Publication Manual of the American Psychological Association* (the fifth edition was published in 2001), others use different sources or develop their own eclectic approach in referencing. Writers of monographs and similar works, in which no particular format is suggested, should choose the style most comfortable for them. Keep in mind that articles generally require a reference list at the end, whereas books include a bibliography and often a listing of references for separate chapters. Whatever the policy of the journal or publishing company, your work should include *only* those references used in the text. When citing your documentation, follow three major principles: *Make it clear, make it complete, and make it accurate.*

Typed double-spaced, references or endnotes may appear alphabetically with the author's last name or in numerical order as cited in the body of the work. Although some style guides recommend the use of ibid., others, such as the University of Chicago, have eliminated the term, along with op. cit. and loc. cit. According to the *Chicago Manual of Style,* the first time that you cite a source, the endnote includes all the publication information for that work and the reference page number if indicated. Subsequent references to a source already cited include the author's last name, an abbreviated title, and the page(s) mentioned.

First Note:

Mary Breckinridge. Wider Neighborhoods: A Story of the Frontier Nursing Service (New York: Harper, 1952), 97.

Subsequent Note:

Breckinridge, Wider Neighborhoods, 162.

Annotations represent an important addition to endnotes because they build on information in the text. They must be not only interesting and relevant but provide clarity to the discussion presented. So, select your annotated material with care and document it as appropriate.

In today's electronic world, you undoubtedly want to know more about extracting information from the Internet and how to reference it properly. Whenever possible, cite the title of the document, the author, address or URL, and the retrieval date. As a writer, you must always seek authoritative data and their sources. Therefore, be certain as well as circumspect that a reference from the Web is up to date and reliable. (See Chapter 5, "Harness the Potential of Computers and the Internet," for further information.)

REFERENCING AND COPYRIGHTED WORKS

Every published work must include the copyright notice to ensure the owner protection. The notice does not have to be included in unpublished material. All authors are protected by federal statute against unauthorized use of their unpublished manuscripts. The Copyright Act of 1976 states that an unpublished work is copyrighted from the moment it appears in tangible form. Until an author finally transfers the copyright, that individual owns the copyright in an unpublished manuscript, and all exclusive rights of the copyright owner are also due to the author of unpublished works.

As an author quoting directly from a published work, you must include the reference citation. It is your responsibility to ascertain whether permission should be sought from the copyright owner. APA style suggests and many journals stipulate that quoted material of 500 words or less does not require permission to reproduce the material. When quoting at length, however, consider appending a footnote with a superscript number, which acknowledges permission from the copyright owner (the copyright owner may require that the credit be given in a particular format). Whether paraphrasing or quoting directly, always credit the source. The key element of this principle is that an author does not present the work of another person as if it were his or her own. When quoting directly, if you find an error in the material, such as a misspelling, then you need to insert the word *sic* in italics and brackets. In this way, you will be protected from assuming accountability for the error.

References for Further Reading

American heritage dictionary of the English language (4th ed.). (2000). Boston: Houghton Mifflin.

American Psychological Association. (2001). *Publication manual of the American Psychological Association* (5th ed.). Washington, DC: Author.

The Chicago manual of style (15th ed.). (2003). Chicago: University of Chicago Press.

Dillard, A. (1990). *The writing life.* New York: HarperCollins.

Fondiller, S. H. (1999). *The writer's workbook.* New York: NLN Press/ Jones & Bartlett.

Goldstein, Norm (Ed.). (2005). *The Associated Press stylebook 2006.* Associated Press.

Gordon, K. E. (1993). *The deluxe transitive vampire: The ultimate handbook of grammar for the innocent, the eager, and the doomed.* New York: Random House.

Gordon, K. E. (1993). *The new well-tempered sentence: A punctuation handbook for the innocent, the eager, and the doomed.* Boston: Houghton Mifflin.

Lambuth, D. (1964). *The golden book on writing.* New York: Viking Press.

Mawson, C. O. Sylvester (Ed.). (1995). *Roget's II: The new thesaurus* (3rd ed.). Boston: Houghton Mifflin.

Merriam-Webster's collegiate dictionary (11th ed.). (2001). Springfield, MA: Merriam-Webster.

Merriam-Webster's collegiate thesaurus. (2001). Springfield, MA: Merriam-Webster.

Merriam-Webster unabridged (3rd ed.). (2003). Springfield, MA: Merriam-Webster.

Siegal, A.M., & Connolly, W. G. (2005). *The New York Times manual of style and usage: Revised and expanded edition.* New York: Three Rivers Press.

Strunk, W., White, E. B., & Angell, R. (2000). *The elements of style* (4th ed.). New York: Longman.

Warriner, J. (1988). *English composition and grammar: Complete course.* Austin, TX: Holt, Rinehart and Winston.

Index

SPRINGER PUBLISHING COMPANY

Teaching Evidence-Based Practice in Nursing

Rona F. Levin, PhD, RN
Harriet R. Feldman, PhD, RN, FAAN, Editors

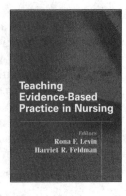

"In their outstanding book, Rona Levin and Harriet Feldman...capture creative approaches to teaching evidence-based practice. This book includes comprehensive and unique strategies for teaching evidence-based practice for all types of learners across a variety of educational and clinical practice settings. The concrete examples of teaching assignments provided in the book bring the content alive and serve as a useful, detailed guide for how to incorporate this material into meaningful exercises for learners. Levin and Feldman's book is a truly wonderful, necessary resource for educators working in all healthcare professional programs as well as clinical settings." —From the Foreword by

Bernadette Mazurek Melnyk, PhD, RN, CPNP/NPP, FAAN, FNAP

Based on the idea that nursing students and nurses at all levels can contribute to the development of a scientific base for nursing practice by critiquing and questioning guidelines, treatments, and outcomes of their own practice, this book examines the ways in which the teaching and learning of evidence-based practice (EBP) occurs. The book provides useful strategies for educators and facilitates the work of faculty to develop curricula that incorporate EBP and the work of nurses implementing EBP in the clinical setting.

Partial Contents

Part I: Setting the Stage

Part II: The Basics of Teaching/Learning Evidence-Based Practice

Part III: Teaching/Learning Evidence-Based Practice in the Academic Setting

Part IV: Teaching/Learning Evidence-Based Practice in the Clinical Setting

2006 · 400pp · 0-8261-3155-7 · softcover

11 West 42nd Street, New York, NY 10036-8002 • Fax: 212-941-7842
Order Toll-Free: 877-687-7476 • Order On-line: www.springerpub.com

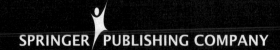

SPRINGER / PUBLISHING COMPANY

Successful Grant Writing

Strategies for Health and Human Service Professionals, Second Edition

Laura N. Gitlin, PhD and Kevin J. Lyons, PhD

Designed for health and human service professionals in academic and practice settings, this book will assist inexperienced grant writers as well as those who have had success but would like to expand their knowledge of grantmanship. The authors provide a framework for understanding the funding world and offer a range of effective strategies and work models for success in obtaining external support. The appendices contain a selection of common questions and their answers and a list of key acronyms.

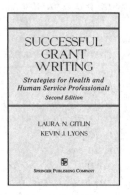

Second Edition Topics include:

- A Research Career Trajectory
- Pilot Research Programs
- What Ideas Are Hot and What Are Not
- The NIH Modular Format
- Elements of a Concept Paper
- Managing the Grant Award

Partial Contents:

Part I: The Perspective of the Funding Agencies • Getting Started • Becoming Familiar with Funding Sources

Part II: The Perspective of the Grantee • Developing Your Ideas for Funding • Learning about Your Institution

Part III: Writing the Proposal • Common Sections of Proposals • Preparing a Budget • Technical Considerations • Strategies for Effective Writing

Part IV: Models for Proposal Development • Four Project Structures • The Process of Collaboration

Part V: Life After a Proposal Submission • Understanding the Review Process • A Case Study

Part VI: Receiving the Grant Award • Managing the Grant Award

2004 · 320pp · 0-8261-9261-0 · softcover

---

11 West 42nd Street, New York, NY 10036-8002 • Fax: 212-941-7842
Order Toll-Free: 877-687-7476 • Order On-line: www.springerpub.com